PSYCH 101

What you didn't learn in nursing school

Written by Kathi Ann Stringer

From the Author that wrote

5150

The One Who Flew Into the Cuckoo's Nest

ISBN: 978-0-6151-9313-7

Website: Kathi's Mental Health Review

http://www.toddlertime.com

Welcome! I am a survivor from the inpatient mental health system and I wrote the book titled, ***"5150 – The One Who Flew Into the Cuckoo's Nest."*** I was treated so badly that I wondered what nursing staff was learning in school. I read everything the local college had to offer on psychiatric nursing. After reading the material I thought, "they sure didn't treat me this way." At that point I decided to dive into a higher level of learning and bought books from the American Psychiatric Association (APA) and also from Aaronson Publishing.

This book is a compilation of my essays over the last ten years and was created from therapeutic models that resonate with actual experience.

A good place to start reading to get the full benefit of this book and understand the terminology would be:

- ***Psych 101 – Unlocking the Secret of Terms***
- ***An Object Relations Approach to Understanding Unusual Behaviors and Disturbances***

Much of my writings were extracted from the work of Glenn O. Gabbard, Margaret Mahler and Sam Vaknin.

For Treaters: Building a therapeutic alliance is imperative to get treatment compliance. This book looks not only at etiology and symptoms in Borderline Personality Disorder (BPD), but also treatment modalities.

Kathi Stringer

About the Author – Kathi Stringer

President and Owner - Companies

Sciatek Industries (left) - 18 years. Gils Western Wear, Grinder Hut, Hair tailors, & Dancetime. Provided parts and engineering for medical, aerospace, electronic, automotive and commercial companies. Knowledgeable in payroll, receivables, engineering, quoting, planning, and quality assurance.

Quality Control - Have written quality control manuals to meet MIL-I-45208A for stringent quality assurance. Have met with agents for quality sourcing and inspection. Have engaged in Corrective Action, Material Review Boards, First Articles and Accountability

Mental Health Experience:

- Advocate for people (staff/clients) in the mental health system
  - People mistreated in psych hospitals
  - People mistreated in out-patient
  - Treaters reaching out for affective treatment modalities
  - Mistreated Providers in contract Mental Health Plans (MHP)
- Member of the Riverside County Western Regional Mental Health Board
- Participant on the Riverside County Quality Improvement Committee (QIC)
- Director for the Far South Region of the California Network of Mental Health Clients (CNMHC)
- Editor of "Performance Improvement Newsletter" (PIN)
- Web owner of Kathi's Mental Health Review http:www.toddlertime.com
- Member of Depression Bipolar Support Alliance of Riverside (DBSA-Riverside)
- Certified to facilitate NAMI Peer-to-Peer courses for consumers
- Author of Mental Health Articles that are Published/Referenced in Research & Teaching Materials

Information for:

- Team Leaders
- Psychologists
- Psychiatrists
- Social Workers
- Registered Nurses (RN)
- Mental Health Workers
- Counselors/Treaters
- Family to Family Mentors
- NAMI Clients/Patients/Consumers

Table of Contents

Introduction to Understanding Theoretical Psychology Terms and Models

Understanding Borderline Personality Disorder (BPD)

<u>Section I – Personal Insight</u>

Section II – Letters/Questions and Understanding

Section III – Clinical Therapeutic Models for Individuals with BPD

On Empathy

Stigma and Mental Illness

Regression & True Infantilism

PSYCH 101

What you didn't learn in nursing school

Letters of Appreciation from helping professionals

Jan 2004, Dear Kathi, I am very much enjoying your paper though I have not finished reading it yet. I have been doing clinical work from an object relations approach with severely emotionally disturbed children in Santa Barbara Ca. since completing my master's thesis in 1987 on transference and countertransference with Borderline Personality Disorder. However, I have not done much research or writing for a while. Recently, I left my full time clinical position and I now coordinate a clinic here in town, part-time. It has given me more time to do more reading and research. The Internet sure is a great way to connect with very knowledgeable people such as yourself on topics we are interested in.

I am particularly impressed with your coverage of Margaret Mahler as I believe her early work has stood the test of time on the important part healthy separation-individuation from the mother plays in healthy/normal personality development. Sincerely, Jim H.

Jan 5, 2003, Thanks for all your hard work you have put into your website http://www.toddlertime.com/dx/borderline

I love the articles relating to transference/countertransference and ways to effectively deal with this empathetically and theraputically. I love that many of the articles provide examples of interactions. It is rare to find information that combines both examples and then the theory to back those examples up. I am a social work student interning on an inpatient psychiatric unit, and have seen many instances of transference (reactions to) and felt it myself. I have luckily had much coursework dealing with transference especially related to trauma, but your site has really helped me understand it further. The articles are written on a level that is complex, but also very very understandable. I have read texts and articles dealing with transference where many terms are used but not defined well (or abstractly), and you define the terms wonderfully. I think many people will find this site helpful, I know I have printed out quite a few articles to read and keep handy. Thank you sooooo much! Meridith

Jan 2, 2003, Dear Ms Stringer, I am putting together a course on self-care for caregivers (Community Support Workers) and I have been searching for material on transference-countertransference. The material on your website is excellent and I would love to incorporate it into our lesson plans. Please advise me as to your permission/copyright policies. Thank you.Bart Begalka

Sprott-Shaw Community College
Coquitlam, B.C.

Sat Nov 16, 2002, Dear Kathi: I have a bachelor's in Psychology with a Mental Health Concentration and have attended a doctoral program in clinical psychology. I am in the process of transferring my credits to a university closer to my home. I have read Otto Kernberg on Borderline and Narcissistic conditions and a few other works on the subject. However, I have found your webpage on Borderline Personality Disorder to be most helpful and a very clear and concise presentation of the problem. I am a women's group facilitator at the local Family Crisis Center for victims of domestic abuse and I have used the information on your website as a much needed refresher course on behaviors usually adopted by individuals who have been traumatized in childhood. Congratulations on this outstanding work. Best regards, Leticia Crawford

Fri Oct 18 2002, Kathi Stringer, Hi! I'm a post-doctorate fellow working with Otto Kernberg and others over at the personality disorder institute associated with Cornell medical college in NY. I'm thinking about updating our website here and making things more useful as we get a lot of questions and requests for basic info that we haven't directly linked through our website before. As I was looking around the web to see what resources are already out there I was impressed by the clear, unbiased, and informative attitude of your site. I was wondering how you would feel about me adding links to your site, resources, and articles (in no way implying that they are our work, of course, and being clear that they will link to another site) when we update our site with more info. What do you think? Meanwhile, I would like to refer people to your site as one possible resource when they have basic questions about Borderline Personality Disorder that they ask by direct email. Before doing this, I wanted to consult with you about it and see if that would in any way make you uncomfortable.

In any case, I also want to just personally let you know that I am impressed by the quality and nature of the info you have on your site. Thanks for being out there! Ken C.

Hello Kathi, I've found your site enormously helpful. I work in a one to one situation with a 14 year old who has been diagnosed BPD. I am this girls' team leader and so I'm searching the net for some info about BPD so that I may best help my client.

I appreciate that you must be snowed under with responses to your site and so I'll understand if you can't respond, however, if you have time I wonder if you could help me.

I'm looking specifically for information about a therapeutic approach to working with adolescents with BPD. I've found all the info about diagnosis and characteristics extremely interesting, now I'd like some more information about treatment. Thank you. Jen Slade

Follow up letter from a helping professional

January 12, 2002, Hello Kathi, I found your response extremely useful. As I said in my original letter, I'd found a great deal of information regarding diagnosis and the characteristics of BPD but very little regarding treatment. Following your response, I was able to put a pack together to distribute to my team and then use this as a base line when we came to care-planning our client. This helped in a number of ways.

Possibly the most significant impact or your work was that it helped my team to understand that it was our client's condition that was making her so difficult to be with at times - and not her.

As professional as my team are, they were finding themselves drawn into petty and destructive arguments, responding negatively to personal insults and generally finding our client difficult to like. This was despite the fact that she was clearly reaching out to them for help and desperately confused by her mixed emotions.

After I introduced your work to them and the BPD pack that I'd put together, the heavy atmosphere in the unit just seemed to lift. The team were able to objectify the condition and this stopped them taking my client's behavior and attitude towards them personally.

The work that had been exhausting and mentally draining before became understandable and stimulating now because we had something with a name, recognizable criteria and also strategies for dealing with it.

The impact for our client was immediate. Because the team felt more confident they responded more positively towards her. Because my client felt less rejected and more accepted, her confidence grew and she was able to develop more positive relationships with each of her team.

This young woman is sixteen next week and we're throwing a surprise party for her. Many of the staff that have worked with her across the years will be there and this is because they have a genuine affection for her.

Prior to her diagnosis we were looking at long term care in a therapeutic setting for this client. Now, because of the work we've been able to do with her, we're moving her towards independence.

Finally, I have been able to pass on the pack I put together, including your response, to other team leaders who have begun working with BPD young people. So, your work has impacted across our organization and on the lives of a number of young people.

Thanks once again for all that you do. Jen Slade

This, as you can discern from posted responses, is a pivotal insight. Are you able to populate this analysis more broadly in professional circles? It's so clinically nonjudgmental and honest and true. It's a great tragedy that people cannot view the world in such terms! I only wish you could dedicated more of your professional energies in this direction. The need is so great and so neglected. A Most Grateful Admirer

Legal - California

I am a public defender in Orange County, with very little prior experience in the mental health arena. I have recently been assigned as the supervising attorney in the mental health unit, and have been trying to gather as much information as possible. Your website has been an invaluable resource and I wanted to thank you for the time and effort you have put into it. Thank you. Lee Blumen

Introduction
to
Understanding
Theoretical Psychology
Terms and Models

Psych 101
Unlocking the Secret of Terms

The Secret Language of the Psychotherapist

Written by Kathi Stringer

Simple talk. It seems like it could be a solution for some of these far-out abstract concepts and a key to understanding them. But sometimes using simple talk makes it hard to grasp the full weight of the concept. So I decided to write a paper on the secret language of psychotherapists to enhance the reader's ability to grasp ideas and enable the reader to explore how these fantastic concepts apply to themselves or to those they love.

Once you get into the meaning of the secret codes, you too can read and communicate with others that also understand the covert codes. Of course, this paper is likely to get longer as individuals request for the breakdown on codes that I forgot to include. So keep an eye out for updated revisions. To help out a bit further, in this paper I will be giving a lot of 'For example." I thought you would appreciate that!

- Affect
- Object Relations
  - Objects
- Splitting
- Object Constancy
- Holding Environment
- Transitional Space
- Transitional Objects
- Transference
  - Psychotic Transference
  - Terrify Transferences
  - Transference Interpretation
    - Clarification
    - Confrontation
    - Interpretation
- Countertransference
  - Countertransference
  - Countertransference Hook
  - Countertransference Reaction
  - Countertransference Hate
  - Countertransference Management
  - Countertransference Punishment
  - Countertransference Gage

- Countertransference Opportunity
- Types of Countertransference

- Projective Identification
  - Projective Identification (anger)
  - Projective Counteridentification (anger)
  - Introjective Identification
    - The Container and the Contained
  - Projective Identification Reviewed
  - Projective Identification Analogy
- The Three Agencies of the Mind
  - Id
    - Primary Process (Id processing)
  - Superego
  - Ego
    - Secondary Process (Ego processing)
- Observing Ego
- Ego Weakness & Strength
- Defense Mechanisms
- Execution Boundary

Affect

Affects are basically the emotions a client displays according to the content they are dealing with. For example, if the appropriate affect that a client should have would be in the range of excitement or enthusiasm, and the client is unresponsive, then the treater may see this as 'flat affect'. Affect is usually appropriate when it matches content. When it does not match, then this is a signal for the treater to examine the situation a little more closely. Laughing inappropriately, lack of emotion from a devastating trauma and etc may be signals for closer exanimation.

Object Relations

Object relations is a term introduced by , Fairburn. He figured that humans were influenced the most by past and current relationships to other individuals as a main force for life. The need for the infant to bond with the primary caretaker was paramount and above the need for food, clothing and shelter. Hence, Object Relations because of the desire to form a Relationship with others is more important then need for sleep, food, shelter and clothing.

Objects

Fairburn viewed objects as internal and external. An internal object is a piece of psychic structure within the personality and external objects are those we relate to externally. For example, an internal object may be a piece of psych structure of how I react to criticism and another internal object may be a piece of psych structure how I react to rejection. Perhaps a few of these internal objects may mobilize and work together as several objects for a whole new affect. If enough objects get together and form a maladaptive recipe, then a person may come off as paranoid and upset. It sounds a bit cold and detached for some to think of parts of an individual and others as objects. However, it serves a purpose to articulate ideas and theory into a cohesive model for exploration and usefulness.

Each object has an affect that accompanies it. Some internal objects seemed to be buried so deep that they seemed closed off and no one can get to them. In a case like this I might say, "closed core internal objects are isolated." It's just a fancy way to say that a person is closed off and can't be reached. But of course, it does say a bit more then that. This is why we use abstract psychic language; it helps get deeper into the process of the mind. Once you get used to it, it can become fun to learn and understand ideas from some of the great thinkers and masters of our time.

Splitting

Now that you got the hang of what an object is, it makes sense to think that these objects can become separated and compartmentalized within the mind. When these internal objects become separated, and one object is not communicating with another object, then we call this '*splitting*'. In other words, the object relationship was split up and fragmented into areas of the mind that do not talk to each other. Lets look at how you would be able to observe if someone is suffering from internal fragmentation. For example, have you ever met anyone that can put you on top of the world one moment and then completely devalue you then next moment? Ever notice how some people cannot see a person as a 'whole continuous person' but rather as devils or as angels? Ever notice how some individuals have all the information but cannot make a rational statement? It's because the mind is fragmented and the internal object relations are 'split' into different compartments.

So what causes a person to split up all these objects into different compartments? Why would anyone choose to be so darn confused and irrational? Hang back, there is an answer for this.

I might get this next point across a little easier if I ask you to pause and remember back if you ever had a time when you couldn't make up your mind. "Should I use the blue paint or the red paint?" or even more stressful, "Should I stay in the marriage or divorce?" Most of the time, the higher the consequences of the decision, the more conflict it will cause within the individual. Conflict is to be ambivalent or of 'two minds' or to become 'split' in the decision making process. Splitting is a defense mechanism that infants and toddlers use to ward off unacceptable anxieties. It is unacceptable to a toddler to withstand unbearable anxiety and as a result, the toddler will split-off what causes the anxiety. A child may be want to be independent but at the same time experience feelings of dependence on the same person. This conflict is unacceptable and the toddler cries in psychic pain from the crisis. On the other hand if a fixated toddler continues to split-off the anxiety caused from the need to be independent, then a chronic dependence would out flank any strivings to become an individual.

Can you see how stress from the consequences of a decision or event may determine how and if the internal objects are fragmented? Ever notice when a person becomes really stressed out that their thought becomes more of a reaction, and at times irrational because it is not well thought out? For an individual that has not moved though the earlier developmental stages, splitting can be a way of life, and their stress will amplify the severity of the split. The more stressed out a person is, the more one hand does not know what the other hand is doing. In therapy, the therapist will try to help the individual become more integrated so that the internal objects can be experienced at the same time without splitting them away from each other. More on this in the 'observing ego' description.

Object Constancy

This is a later stage of object relations theory, and overlapping the defense of splitting. It begins to take hold when mother is reliable and keeps returning and emotionally refueling the child. For instance, a toddler may achieve greater and greater distances from mother, but when anxiety in the child takes over, the child will return to mother to refill with her 'essence'. But if the mother is not available upon return, and it happens often, the child may begin to get clingy and afraid to leave thinking he will lose her while he is away.

If mother is 'good enough', and present most times when a child returns (rapprochement), the child begins to develop a mental security of an image that mother is emotionally present, even while away. Some children (and adults) whose mental security is not completely developed may use items like security blankets or stuffed animals to help with the 'transition'. These items are called 'transitional objects'.

When a person is able to internalize a 'constant' representation of another person, even when that person is gone, then that person has developed *object constancy*. Object constancy comes from stability and trust. For example, if a child's parent is radical, invalidating and mistrusting, then the child did not experience stability. The child lived on a roller-coaster without any point of reference for a 'normal' life. Or, if a treater threatens to ban the client for acting-out (yelling) then, the treater fails to become a constant object in the mind of the client. This is harmful because the client may feel less secure out of the presence of the treater, since when leaving the treater, the client becomes afraid he will lose the treater. Out of sight, out of mind. However, if the treater were available, constant and reliable, and able to listen, validate, teach and provided a new positive experiences, then this would have helped the client develop object constancy by modifying his old core beliefs.

Holding Environment

Love this term and was coined by relations theorist named Winnicott. Winnicott figured that by providing structure and a consistent venue for the client, then a sense of safety and trust would develop from the 'holding' experience. The *holding environment* would set the stage and allow the client to cry, vent, and regress in transference (go back to an earlier stage of functioning). For example a client may feel 'held' with structured appointments, phone contact for crisis, and follow up from the treater looking in on the client's welfare, and overall taking on a sort of parental function as outlined in the infant/mother dyad.

Transitional Space

In this 'in between' space the client and the treater can take on assigned roles and act them out much like a child will take on roles when playing. For example, when a client is acting-out toward a treater because of feelings aroused from childhood abuse, the client can then been seen as assigning the treater the role of the abusive parent. It is in this space that old feelings, thoughts and behaviors are awakened for modification…to make a transition. For example, the treater may behave much more consistent and less punitive then the real parent, and this experience will provide a space for transition.

Transitional Object

A transitional object is an object that helps the small child process through a transitional stage in life. Mostly, when the primary care taker is not available, a child may imbue an object with a symbolic meaning to represent mother to help with feelings of insecurity. The object can be a diaper, soft blanket, bottle or other similar item. It usually takes the form of something soft and perhaps the smell of mother.

The object is important to the small child since the child believed that they created it and they full control of the object. It is transitional because the child entered into the beginning of becoming an individual and separate from his mother. The transitional object helped comfort and soothed the child from maternal separations.

As adults, some individuals have not completely separated and are still attached to transitional objects. For example, a patient may view her pills as transitional object because they represent a link to her compassionate and caring doctor. Taking a pill would represent being empathically held and nurtured. Some adults still use infantile transitional objects from childhood. Others may view their therapist 'as' the transitional object, which makes it a bit more difficult for the client to have control over the object.

Transference

Freud came up with this term and it has been used widely ever since. Transference is basically the 'transference' of love or hate from past relationships onto the treater. A psychodynamic treater may try and 'grow' or 'develop' transference between them. Think of it as stirring the pot to see what comes up. For example a treater might make a slight criticism aimed at the client, and then the client may blow up in the treater's face. Way over kill. But in the client's mind, her mother was very critical as she was growing up, and then the slight criticism from treater came at a moody time for the client and was the fuse to ignite the bomb. Wham. Once the treater recovers, the treater would try to figure out exactly what that was all about. In this case, can you see how the client's hate of criticism was transferred from a past relationship with mother and onto treater? This is how transference can be a handy tool to figure out how the client relates to life.

Psychotic Transference

In the example above, with guidance the client may realize that the treater is not really their mother and that the harsh criticisms came from mother. Now in a psychotic transference, the client believes that the treater is the critical mother and none of the material is transferred from the past onto the treater. Basically, that the treater 'is' the client's mother.

Terrifying Transferences.

A client may be afraid to open up and trust a treater. A client may be terrified of what may come as a result of the formed transference. For example, if the client regresses and begins to depend on the treater, then of course the client with abandonment issues will be freaked out at the thought the treater may reject them. This could be viewed as a terrifying transference. Transference because the trust hoped for from a maternal relationship was 'transferened' to the treater; assigned to the treater to play the role as the good-enough mother. A client may resist forming this sort of transference with the treater since the thought of getting dumped and thrown out is too 'terrifying'

Transference Interpretation

This is a handy little tool to give insight into thought patterns that leads at times to behavior. The treater tries to 'grow' a transference between them, so a treater will have some clues as to how the client relates to life, and how the personality works with interpersonal material from self, others and the environment.

Clarification

The treater takes the material (transference) that has formed in the therapeutic relationship and seeks to clarify what is going on in the transference that has developed between client and treater. That is the whole goal of getting a transference going anyway, to get something going to work with. Once the treater has something in their hands, they seek to get a handle on exactly what it is they are looking at. A treater may ask a client if they are looking at the situation correctly, according to the way the clients sees things. If yes, then the treater goes to step two.

Confrontation

Once the treater figures out what is going on in the transference, then the client may get the boom lowered on them. Confronted. Once confronted, and things get hashed out between them, and a sort of agreement is made, then it goes to step three.

Interpretation

Once clarified and confronted, and the time is right, then a treater may interpret their take on why a client behaves the way they do. Of course, the treater first should make every opportunity to get the client to figure out what is going on for themselves. In this way, the client can 'own' the results and insight a little better then if it was handed to them verbally from the treater. In some cases though, the client will never get it and the treater will have to spell it out because no amount of guidance will lead the client to where the treater is leading them.

Countertransference

This is a term first used by Freud and has taken on different properties throughout the century. I am mainly interested right now in describing the current meaning of countertransference as illustrated by Gabbard [5] et al (APA)

Countertransference

Countertransference is transference from the client 'colored' with the unresolved issues of the treater. For example, a client my transfer hate from a critical father onto the treater. The treater feels this transfer of critical hate, and since this hate from the client is not deserved and distorted, then may raise some unfinished feelings inside the treater. The treater is now experiencing a combination of the feelings from the client in 'addition' to their own feelings activated by the client.

Sometimes countertransference can be a tool that the treater can use that can act as a gage or barometer (Gabbard) [5] to measure what is going on inside the client. For example, if the treater is feeling a lot of anxiety from the client's material, then the same thing is likely going on inside the client. If the treater feels anxious from countertransference, then using countertransference as a gage, the treater can get an idea of how the client is feeling at the moment; anxious too.

Countertransference Hook

Of course every treater reacts according to what is said to them. What might bother one treater may not bother another treater. So every treater has their own countertransference hook, depending upon their unique personality (Gabbard) [5]. Sometimes a client can tell if a treater has been hooked by their facial or body expression.

Countertransference Reaction

This happens when a treater reacts to the countertransference. This could take the form of giving out a maladaptive and untruthful diagnosis that could hurt the client, or drift off daydreaming and ignore the client, or cancel appointments, or end session abruptly, or threaten to ban them for the practice (execution boundary), or raise their fees, or feel sexually attracted toward the client, or have a desire to do heroic endeavors to protect the client, or… I think you get the idea.

Countertransference Hate

For example, if the client enjoys beating animals, then hearing this can trigger a hate toward the client.

Countertransference Management

A skillful treater knows the importance of having countertransference management. It can prevent the treater/client relationship from going beyond repair. For example, a mental health worker (MH) might say to a client, "Get back on the other side of the Red Line!" A client may react after perceiving this as a harsh tone by saying, "Or what???" At this point if the MH worker does not manage their countertransference, they may say, "Or you will go into seclusion and restraints!" Which fosters hate toward the treater in the client. On the other hand with countertransference management a treater could say, "The reason we need you to stay on this side of the Red Line is so that you will be safer on the unit. We care about your safety and this is way we need you to be on this side of the Red Line." This would come across as much more thoughtful with a warm personal regard.

Countertransference Punishment

A treater that is fed up might secretly wish the client would succeed in killing themselves so the treater can escape the problem of having to deal with the client. With this thought a treater may withdraw and become aloft and withhold redirection to keep the client from killing themselves. Or, for another example, if staff on an inpatient unit would put a client into seclusion as a form of a penalty, this is also called countertransference punishment. This is illegal since a client can't be put into seclusion unless they are a danger to themselves, others, or destroying community property. However, even though a client does not meet any of this criteria, staff has been known many times to put a client into seclusion for 'convenience of staff.'

Countertransference Gage

Countertransference if used correctly can be used as sort of a gage to measure what is going on inside of the client. For example, it a treater feels like his veins are about to pop out of the side of his neck, then the feelings generated inside of the treater will give an indication of what is going on inside of the client. Ever notice how when two people are yelling at each other that both of them are angry and frustrated? The same with countertransference because it acts as sort of an internal mirror of what is going on inside the client. This is why it is called a countertransference gage. The treater, by measuring their own discomfort they can get an idea of how uncomfortable the client is feeling. A handy little tool if used correctly.

Countertransference Opportunity

Love this one. When a client is ticking off the treater, the client usually expects that which has always been given....to get it back in their face, or to get something back anyway. Yet, if the treater viewed countertransference as an opportunity to answer back in a less hurtful tone, then the treater was able to offer a therapeutic experience for the client.

Types of Countertransference

So far the type of countertransference I have been talking about is anger in the treater from the client. There are all kinds of different countertransferences though. For example, a narcissist countertransference is working when the client idolizes the treater and the treater promotes it and distorts it...."I am the all good treater, all knowing and all good" type of thing. Or a client may present as more helpless then they truly are and the treater becomes the 'rescuer' of the client. The treater may then feel obligated use heroic efforts to save the client repeatedly and this creates misery in the treater, which can change from countertransference-rescuer to countertransference-hate. The point is, countertransference comes in many forms and not just from anger.

Projective Identification (3 Levers)

This term was coined and introduced by Marie Klein. However not much was elaborated on its significance. The term at times takes on different meaning according to the author. Ogan helped resolve getting a grip on this extremely difficult concept by dividing the dynamic into three levers as outlined below. This is the current modern concept as published by the APA, Gabbard et al, and the Minniger Clinic of Kansas.

In the examples below, I am referring to anger being projected. But remember, as internal objects of the mind, any object, or cluster of objects can be split-off and projected. Similar, as there can be many types of countertransference feelings in the treater, many different types of objects can be projected onto the treater from the client. A projected object is not isolated to only anger, yet anger does seem to be the most frequent projection to deal with.

Projective Identification (anger / Lever 1)

This can be related to pushing the treater's 'buttons'. After a client is able to find the treater's weak spots (a countertransference hook), the client can then push a treater's buttons as a way to gain control over the treater.

Think of a client that is dealing with unresolved anger from childhood and the treater said something that ticked off the client. The get even, the client may start looking for 'hot spots' in the treater and once found, a client can push a treater's hot buttons. A client may think, "you made me upset, so now I'm going to get even and get you upset, to show you what it feels like." See how there is an element of control here? To get even, the client needs get control and 'make' the treater feel just as bad or worse then the client.

Projective Identification is different then countertransference due to one single element. Projective Identification has a 'force' behind it. A client is projecting (forcing) a part of themselves (identity) onto the treater. It's all about force and the strength of that force. The bigger the hot button in the treater, the stronger the force. Control, control and control.

So far in this first lever, a client is projecting anger onto the treater. At this point nothing will happen unless the treater identifies with the projected object of anger. If this happens, we go to stage two, projective counteridentification.

Projective Counteridentification (anger / Lever 2)

At this point a treater has identified with the projected object of anger. In other words, the client has successfully found the treater's hot buttons and pushed them and the treater is really ticked off. A treater will usually feel so ticked off, that they are no longer themselves. <u>It is as if an alien force has taken them over</u>. A treater at this point may feel very miserable and want to dump the client. The anger that now resides in the treater is a product of the treater's repressed anger (the hot button) in 'addition' to the anger projected from the client. It is quite a lot to handle.

Introjective Identification (Lever 3)

This third lever is where the magic comes in. Of course for this lever to work, the treater must be working to identify what has happened in the first two levers. This may take some time.

A client may expect the treater to react the same as other persons, usually from past childhood relationships. A client may expect to get dumped and abandoned just like in the past. And in the client's mind, this proves they were right all along. The client may think, "See, I am bad and I can be cast out. You were lying to me all along and you are just as rejecting as everyone else, and just as hurtful." And then the cycle repeats, unless a treater is able to get a grip and use these two tools:

The Container and the Contained

A treater can act as a container for the projected objects (Gabbard) [1] from the client. Note, this is far different then the treater acting as a sponge and absorbing the vile projections. Rather, the Container in the treater acts like a pot to hold that projected anger. Once the anger is in the pot (container) a treater can identify and work with the anger (contained).

Now that the anger has been contained carefully within the treater, the treater can skillfully detoxify, metabolize and modify the object of anger. For example a treater might not react badly to the client and rather more calmly, emphatically, and totally different then what was expected. A treater may act in a structured, soothing and continuous affect. This of course modifies the client's perception of reality.

Once the treater has acted as a container, and contained the object, and has further modified that object, the treater can now offer something more manageable back to the client for assimilation. Of course the treater 'cannot make' the client accept what is offered. The client may just blow it off. But usually if what the treater's offers is attractive for the client, the client will then take in and assimilate the modified object of anger. The returned anger from the treater is less harsh and defused.
This third step is magic because a treater is able to modify that which was 'closed' off or hidden inside the client. The treater, like a wizard that is able to execute magic, can change the client can change the client by offering a new and better internal world for the client. Sort of like cutting down on the inside pain by responding much different then abusive past relationships and offering a new role model.

Projective Identification Reviewed

Lever One, Projective Identification:
A client splits-off and projects (with force) an object (anger) into the treater via the countertransference hook.

Lever Two, Projective Counteridentification:
The treater has identified with the projected object (anger) and has taken it in. The treater feels as though not themselves. Like an alien force has taken them over.

Lever Three, Introjective Identification:
When skillfully used, a treater can act as a container and contain the object (anger), and modify it into something (a modified introject) that is much more attractive for the client. The client may now identify and assimilate the offered introject, hence we now have Introjective identification.

Projective Identification Analogy

The following is an analogy of Transference, Countertransference, Countertransference Management, Projective Identification, Projective Counteridentification, Introjective Identification, and the Container and the Contained. The analogy is a spoof off Star Trek with the Client acting as the mysterious new Life Form and the USS Enterprise and Crew acting as the Treater.

Star Date: 2002 – Captain's Log 4231: Recording of ship's transcripts of an unknown life form in uncharted space.

Sulu: "Captain, there appears to be an unknown Life Form ahead."

Captain Kirk: "Put is on screen Sulu *[Treater visual assessment]* and Spock, report."

Spock: "I am picking up strange readings, it appears that we are being scanned Captain."
[client developing a transference]

Sulu: "The Life Form is beginning to change shape Captain, and it appears to be threatening.
[Client as developed an transference consisting of anger toward the Treater]

Captain: "Reverse engines, full impulse power, Scotty, give me all ya got" *[countertransference reaction]*

Spock: "Captain, we are still being scanned, and the life form now resembles lethal anti-matter that could destroy this sector if it should converge with our dilithium crystals housed in the engine room.

Captain Kirk: "Raise shields and go to Red Alert!" *[countertransference management]*

Spock: "Captain, the Life Form has fired a Probe and will make contact right about...now!"

SHIP SHAKES
[attempt at projective identification]

Captain Kirk: "Damage Report!"

Sulu: "Our shields holding Captain."

Spock: "The Life Form has fired another probe, and scanners show a slight configuration from the last probe, and will make contact....now!"

SHIP SHAKES
[another attempt at projective identification as the Client is looking for a weak spot in the Treater]

Sulu: "Shields down 20% and auxiliary power is ready to go on-line Sir."

Spock: "Captain, the Life Form has fired another probe and it is configured once again. Probe should make contact about ....."

FLASH, AND BURST OF BLUE LIGHT

*****The Probe has made contact with the ship***
[projective counteridentification]

Captain: "What's happening"

Spock: "The Probe as penetrated our shields and I detect a strong surge of energy from the Probe taking command of the ship's computer."

[projective counteridentification is complete, the Client will now attempt to control the treater.]

Captain Kirk: "Spock, what was that? What happened!?" I need answers and I need them fast!"

Spock: "Sir, the Probe has been configured to get past our shields and has attached itself to the haul of the ship. The Probe has interfaced with our ships communications node and is reassigning our electronic parameters to that of the host Life Form that launched the Probe."

Captain: "Spock! Is there anything we can do? Think of something!"

Spock: "Captain, most of the Ship's database is infected and the control of the Ship is being redirected by the probe. Life support is at risk and the ship's energy seems to dwindling away. <u>It is if an alien force has taken us over."</u>
[confirmation of projective counteridentification onto the Treater]

Ship's Computer: LIFE SUPPORT WARNING: "Ship's oxygen 72% and decreasing"
[effects of projective counteridentification is miserable for the Treater]

Captain: "Spock! Talk to me! Think of something, we don't have much time!"

Spock: "My analysis confirms a power surge in communication node C-32 on deck four from the alien probe. We can reroute the Ship's command and reinitialize the contaminated database to contain the projected energy radiating from the probe. It seems Captain, that the probe is receiving instructions from the host Life Form."

Captain: "Okay Spock, reinitialize and retake command of the Ship"
[Treater has identified and contained the project object]

Sulu: "Sir, the Life Form shows signs of distress. Should we follow procedures as outlined in the Prime Directive?"

Captain: "You are absolutely right Sulu. Spock, can you send the Probe back to the host Life Form with a message of good will from Star Fleet?"

Spock: "Yes Captain, now that we have contained the Probe we are able to detoxify and metabolize the opposing forces within the Probe. We can modify the Probe's circuits and offer something more attractive to the Life Form."

Captain: "Do it Spock. The quicker, the better."

Scotty: "Captain, the modified Probe is ready to be launched. Shall I proceed?"
[the projected object from the projective identification onto the Treater has been detoxified, modified and made into something more manageable for the Client.]

Captain: "Proceed Scotty. Spock, target the Life Form and the reuptake of the Probe. Record activity into Ship's log for Star Fleet.

THE USS ENTERPRISE FIRES THE ALIEN'S PROBE BACK TOWARD THE HOST LIFE FORM FOR POSSIBLE ASSIMILATION.
[once modified, the Treater can offer a more attractive object to the Client for assimilation]

Spock: "It appears Captain that the Life Form, has accepted and assimilated the Probe that we modified back into its core structure." [intorjective identification, the Client accepted the modified object]

Sulu: "CAPTAIN! Look! The Life Form is changing! It somehow looks less threatening...and...and...it looks....happy Sir?!"

Spock: "It appears Sir, that you have helped give birth to new Life Form. Even though it cannot communicate, which is puzzling, it does seem to have a bit of...humanness?
[the Client can now see the world as a better place in which to live]

Captain Kirk: "I think you are right about that Spock. Attention bridge, since we are going to be in this sector of space for a while, design and implement a system to address additional Probes from the Life Form. Perhaps over time and with each Probe we modify, we can offer a bit more of humanity to a race that does not understand us. "

Spock: "Captain, what should we call the project?"

Captain Kirk: "Spock...lets call it......First Contact"

Star Date 200[*] -- Captain's Log 4232 The threatening Live Form was able to penetrate our shields with a projected Probe. The crew was contain and modify the Probe and fire it back to the Life From. First contact was successful.

The Three Agencies of the Mind

Freud theorized (Hall) [8] that the mind works from a system governed by an executive agency, the *ego*. The other two agencies are the *id* (infant) and the *superego* (parent). This in its self suggests the mind is fragmented. Over time, and with experience with what works and what doesn't work, the mind is able to act more as a team unit.

Id

The Id is the demanding part of the mind. It acts on getting its needs met immediately and impulsively. The id remains infantile in character throughout life (Hall) [8] with traits that are demanding, irrational, asocial, selfish and pleasure-loving. The id lacks organization compared to the ego and superego, and does not change with time. More interesting, the id cannot be modified be experience since it has no contact with the external world.

Primary Process (Id processing)

Primary Process (Hall) [8] comes out of the Id. It is raw impulses without any rationalization. For example, if I suggest a person acts impulsively out of the Primary Process, then I am suggesting a person is acting irrational and their thought is without consideration from the demands of reality. For example, Primary Process thinking my be, "I got to go pee" and then just pee on the spot, and not wait until going to the restroom.

Superego

The superego is the ideal agency of the mind. It is the moral or judicial branch of the personality, the inner critic. It seeks unrealistic perfection rather then pleasure or reality. The superego develops its moral code out the ego though absorption of discipline from parents, schoolteachers, religious agents and authority figures. The Superego will bug you to be the 'perfect' human being according to the rewards or punishment you got when growing up. Consequences from discipline give rise to the formation and incorporation for what is bad, good, moral, and immoral. It the Superego that will lay the guilt on you.

The superego formed out of the child's wishes for love. Not being loved means an unloving mother that withholds food, emotional soothing and other vital life necessities. For the superego to be effective it must exercise the same power as the parents as the child gets older.

Ego

Even though this guy is in the 'middle' I saved him for last. The ego is the decision maker, making transactions between the self and cultural reality, controlling and governing the id and the superego while maintaining socially accepted behavior with the external world. The ego acts as a negotiator between 3 pressures. The Id wants its way, the Superego usually wants it much different, and then there are the demands on what is acceptable in the world. .i.e. reality. For example, a person out hiking has to go pee, the Id thinks, "Pee right now!" the Superego thinks, "not until you get home!" and the Ego thinks that both are unreasonable and checks out the path for a hidden place to go pee. What happened here is that the Ego delayed the Id's impulse to go right away, and negotiated with the Superego not to wait forever, and dealt with reality to find a hidden place as not to attract attention as culturally discouraged. . The ego is basically an executive agency (Hall) [8] of the system dedicated to thinking and problem solving. The growth of the ego comes from reality testing which will improve perception, thinking, memory and action. As function of the ego develops it can perceive the external world with greater precision and accuracy, and of course, make better choices.

Secondary Process (Ego processing)

Out of the Ego comes thought that is more rational. It is the Ego's job to check with all the demands of the mind. Each part of the agency has it own agenda. When the Ego checks with each agency and with reality, it is performing a Secondary Process. Secondary Process (Hall) [8] comes from contemplating, experience and thinking things out and getting in touch with all fragments of the mind. So if I say something like, "His thought process resembles more of the impulsive Primary Process, rather then the more rational Secondary Process. Sort of an insult to some by referring to them a main a Primary Process thinker....meaning life has not taught them very much.

Observing Ego

This guy keeps track of what is going on once a person begins to develop it. For example, Nancy and her treater are barking at each other and nothing is getting resolved. The treater has usually developed an 'observing ego' to keep track what is going on, to whom does what. With clients the feelings in the treater get aroused. In this example, a treater is getting angry at Nancy for her remarks. Because of the wonderful training

of the treater, she will check with the observing ego and search for what is 'really' going on. Perhaps the observing ego might offer that Nancy is using her anger as a defense because the treater is getting to close to some walled off feelings and it is making Nancy uncomfortable and defensive.
Another example could be when two people are fighting and nothing is getting resolved. If one person has a developed observing ego, then that person may 'fall back and regroup", and try and approach the fight from a different perspective. The observing ego would be like a third person looking down from above and 'objectively' keep track of what is going on. The observing ego is more detached from the 'feelings', which gives it a base to be more logical.
It takes some practice to develop an observing ego, but it is well worth it.

Ego Weakness & Strength

Ego strength enables a person to withstand stress while deciding on what to do with the problem. If a person caves to stress, and does not weigh out each area of the Id, Superego and Reality, then there is a weakness in the Ego. For example, lets say a couple are getting frustrated in a conversation. One person finally became so overwhelmed with stress that they told the other person to 'stick it' and stormed off. In this case, the person became vulnerable to impulsive action as the stress became intolerable. The anger of the Id overtook the strength of the Ego and won. The idea is to develop Ego strength as life moves on.

Ego strength also helps the mind become less fragmented. For example, part A of the mind may have strong tendency to see a person as all bad. Part B sees the person as all good. There is a conflict going on here. If a person had weak ego strength, they would just give into side A or to side B. It is the Ego's job to be strong enough to withstand the conflict and see areas of gray in the person. The higher the 'stress' the higher the Ego strength needs to be to maintain a level head.

Defense Mechanisms

The mind uses defenses to protect its self from injury or stress. These defenses have been giving names to help identity what is going on and get to the bottom of it. Persons with greater Ego strength tend to use more advanced defenses then a person with regressed or weak Ego strength. The names of some of these defenses are listed below (Stringer) [7].

- Projection
- Denial
- Suppression
- Regression
- Rationalization

- Intellectualization
- Reaction Formation

Execution Boundary

This is the most dreaded of all boundaries in therapy. Some treater's will bring up the Execution Boundary (Stringer) [6] to blackmail the client into behaving a different way. For example a treater might say, "if you yell at me one more time, I will ban you from my practice" or "if you don't try harder, I will not see you anymore." Usually when a treater is not as qualified, they will tend to use the threat of the Execution Boundary, which in most case can have a devastating effect on therapy. The client might think, "See, I was right all along, I am bad, I can be cast out, and you are 'never' to be trusted." Then the trust issue is scraped out and everything gets set back…again.

References:

1. Integrated Treatment of Borderline Personality Disorder - Glen O. Gabbard, M. D. - Video Lecture / APA Series

2. Diagnostic and Statistical Manual of Mental Disorders DSM-IV-TR - American Psychiatric Association (APA)
[Book Link]

3. Cognitive-Behavioral Treatment of Borderline Personality Disorder - Linehan
[Book Link]

4. I Hate You, Don't Leave Me - Jerold Kreisman, M.D., Hal Straus
[Book Link]

5. Countertransference Issues in Psychiatric Treatment - Glen O. Gabbard, M.D.
[Book Link]

6. The Execution Boundary and Borderline Hatred - Kathi Stringer
[Page Link]

7. An Object Relations Approach to Understanding Unusual Behaviors and Disturbances - Kathi Stringer
[Page Link]

8. A Primer of Freudian Psychology - Calvin S. Hall
[Book Link]

An Object Relations Approach to Understanding Unusual Behaviors and Disturbances

What an enormous sweep! A tour-de-force!
Samuel Vaknin, Ph.D.

Written by Kathi Stringer
Released June 28, 2003
Revision A April 20, 2006 (SMP to SLP)

Dedication

To my good friend, Sam Vaknin.
No matter the obstacles, he's got heart. Sam is a true survivor.

Objective

To explain pathology disturbances and their manifestations entrenched early in child development. These disturbances may manifest as personality disorders (Axis II) such as ***borderline personality*** disorder, ***narcissistic personality*** disorder or, pathology disturbances may manifest as ***obsessive***, chronic and unusual behaviors such as ***transvestitism***, *infantilism, autism* and pathological ***passiveness,*** or ***reactive attachment*** disorder. We will see how the variables the child brings to the table, i.e.... his temperament, intelligence and etc, combined with his journey, assimilation and resolution though these critical milestones embedded in child development will shape the child's sense of self.
We will explore how integration of the self is developed though oscillation of frustration and satisfaction. We will see how the good-enough mother regulates and modulates the infant's anxiety to promote growth or on the flipside, maladaptive defensives. We will examine the difficult questions that appear elusive and grounded into the unknown. We will address the haunting questions of 'why' and offer components to build structures so the equation may be articulated in terms that provide understanding and relief. We will attempt to connect to the "ahhhhhh...." The 'ah' can provide a sense of identity, of awareness and diminish guilt. The 'ah' can provide a beginning point for growth that was lost in the abyss of the unconsciousness.

Source

This paper has applied widely accepted models grounded in object relations. The main source of this material was lifted from the observations, conclusions and scholarly work of Margaret Mahler and her dedicated collages. Mahler had secured grants that funded a major project that setup a natural framework to observe mothers interactions with their children as they moved through their developmental phases. Mahler's carefully arranged setting for observations (one-way glass) included an infant's room and a transitional hallway that led into the toddler's room. *"Thus, we had an observational situation that provided many opportunities for the observation of mother-infant separations and reunions. [4]* Mahler arranged experiments to measure the infants and toddlers frustration toleration when separated from mother at different time intervals. Data was collected based on the degree of attunement in which mother and infant were able to communicate. Mahler and her collages observed passive separations as well as deliberate separations, i.e. when mother would leave the room for an interview with staff.

Terminology

Through observations Mahler et al hypothesize that satisfactory relationships (object relations) with the primary caretaker are parliament to (above the need for) food, clothing and shelter. Object relations is a powerful language. Since I will be using this language, I will review its basic foundation.

Object Relations

An internal *object* is a piece of psychic structure within the personality whereas external objects are those we relate to externally. Object relations theorists explain that an internal object that is affected by an external object will modify perception within the structure of the self (Interactions with our environment alters our perception of reality through *validation – strengthens our perception* – or – *modification – alters our perception*). There is a mix of object relating with the mind and environment. The manner external objects (family, cousins, friends, dog, cat, tree..etc) are organized in the environment affects the internal objects (psychic structures) through the modification of perception within the self. For example and to simplify,

> The instructor (object) disciplined two of his students (objects). One student came from a military home and one from a street gang. The military student thanked his instructor for the discipline, whereas the street gang student clinched his fist.
>
> Through investigation we may discover that the military student viewed discipline as 'being noticed' and the discipline validated his family relationship with his idolized father. We could say that the military student had a strict father-son relationship (strict object relations) that modified his perception of his teacher, as

the 'good' teacher (the good object). Or we could say in more abstract object relation terms "Because of his strict object relations the student was able to identify with the ridged and demanding object without overwhelming frustration." It is extremely helpful to work with objects when observing, constructing, deconstructing, analyzing and understanding the network of the mind.

Let's briefly talk about the 'splitting'. As we have learned, an internal object is a piece of psyche structure. Therefore it makes sense that these objects can split-off or clump together to form complex objects or mechanisms (defense mechanisms). The formation of complex objects form how an individual relates, or reacts to self or the environment. Let's view how a toddler 'splits' his internal objects as a defense to save his relationship with mother.

Mother disciplines her child by placing him in 'time-out.' The child is brewing with anger and begins screaming. A different adult enters the time-out to investigate and soothe the child. The child's mood escalates into a lock-in rage. This appears as a mystery. However, through object relations it is reasonable to hypothesize that the toddler viewed mother as the 'all good object' and in order to preserve the all good relationship with mother, the child 'split' the investigating adult as 'all bad' *instead* of mother. In other words, the toddler took out his rage on someone else other then the all-good maternal love object.

Object relations' theorists often times debate the 'exact' formula that applies to a word or complex. In some cases a theorist's will debate as to whether an object is introjected 'onto' or 'into' the target. Theorists can have slightly different views. For example: "selfobject, internal object, and introject" (Kohut, Winnicott, Mahler, Kernberg, Bion & Fairbairn) to name a few, can be used loosely or with tight restriction depending on the author. However, for this paper, the differences are slight and we will not delve into the different arguments that beg for further clarification. To do so would be beyond the scope of this work.

Lets clarify another word. Libido. We are not talking so much about sex drive here as we are talking about the *force of life* (Vaknin). When we are talking about "libidinal separations from mother," we are talking about the child's separation from mother's essence of love, or perhaps the child's feelings of abandonment due to being libidinally separated.

Topographical Model

Object relations are a *supplement* to psychodynamic theory to understand current behaviors and relationships deriving from the mother-infant dyad. The emphasis of this work is framed in Margaret Mahler's et al developmental phases, primarily the emerging *Separation –Individuation phase out of* the powerful regressive force of the *Symbiotic phase.* Settlage states "*Separation-individuation theory places the primary love object, the mother, in the central position in human development.*" [1] We will see how the separation-individuation dynamic acts as the 'training wheels' for the infant to move beyond the delusional and blissful state of 'oneness with creation,' (fantasy-regressive) into an independent 'oneness with self' (reality-mature).

Scope

I. Nature vs. Nurture

II. Overview of Mahler's Developmental Stages

III. In Depth on Rapprochement Behaviors and Complexes

IV. Separation-Individuation Disturbances

V. Symbiotic Libidinal Pull (SMP) and Manifestations

VI. Conclusion

I. Nature vs. Nurture

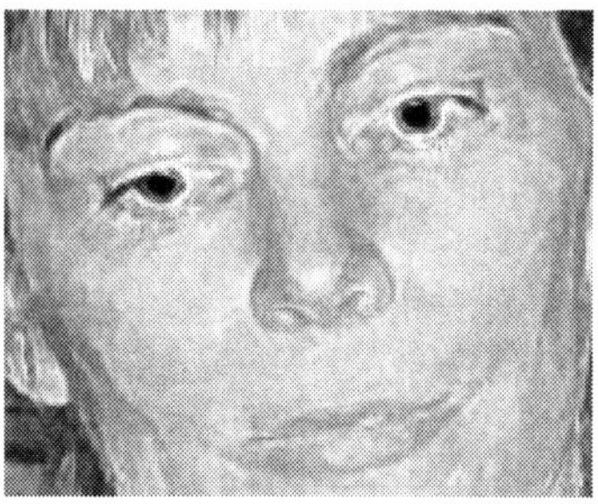

The objective of this material is not to project absolute responsibility on the parent or the child. Each contributes to the evolving development of the self. Settlage states, "*The child's contribution includes the innate givens, such as temperament, tendency toward activity or passivity, affective intensity, anxiety tolerance, and the intelligence and fantasy potential* [1]. Rather, this material is offered to bring a sense of 'awareness' to explain with reasonable, and accepted models how the *product* of child pathology is derived from the reverberation of nature vs. nurture. Many individuals are in constant bewilderment as to why they are different, or chronically neurotic, or lacking identity, or defective because they are seeking maternal equilibrium, or self-destructive, or vacillating with confusion without any 'center' or 'point of reference.'

The question of nature vs. nurture is important because with good road maps we can analyze and reconstruct psychopathology with objectively rather then projecting inappropriate blame. For instance, insight would be helpful for these questions: "I had the perfect childhood, what's wrong with me?" or "I know that I was abused, but why can't I get over it?" or "My brothers and sisters turned out okay, why do I feel so different?

These questions and more will be addressed as we reconstruct the dynamics of nature vs. nurture as observed in infants and toddlers by Margaret Mahler and her collogues. We will also investigate attachment, bonding, trauma and object phenomena as explain by object relations theorists and psychodynamic theorists.

II. Overview of Mahler's Developmental Stages

Mahler's Stages can be outline as thus:

- Normal Autistic Phase (about 1 month)
- Symbiotic Phase (1 / 4-5 months)
- Separation-Individualization Phase (four subphases - begins about 4 to 5 months)
    - Differentiation (4-5 / 10-12 months)
    - Practicing (10-12 / 16-18 months)
    - Rapprochement (16-18 / 22-24 months)
    - On the Way to Object Constancy (22-24 / about 3 years...)

The two forerunners of Mahler's 4-part Separation-Individualization phase are the *normal autistic phase* quickly followed by the powerful *symbiotic phase*. The autistic phase is more or less a 30-day period in which the mother's duties lend more toward the physical care of her infant. Think of the autistic phase as sort of waiting period until the infant gains a slight perception of the environment. During the autistic phase the infant's perception is *one-with-self,* a sort of closed psychological membrane (less mother - therefore autistic). Then, though an accumulation of experiences with mother, there is a shift out of *one-with-self* into *one-with-mother*, the symbiotic phase. Now materializes another confusing word, narcissism. Narcissism at this stage of development is a sense that one is more powerful then one really is. This is natural because mother is perceived as a more *powerful extension* of the infant. It may be helpful to view the symbiotic phase as infant-mother = infant-powerful = narcissistic infant (healthy narcissism). As you can see, viewed from the infant's perspective, this is a natural progression, and healthy toward a normal development.

Normal Autistic Phase – 4 Weeks

At birth the physiological event was dramatic and witnessed. However, the newborn's psychological awareness outside his autistic orbit, his awareness of 'other' as separate being does not exist at this point. The primary nature of his inborn instincts are his discharge of tension from thirst, hunger, elimination, temperature regulation and other physiological requirements that are maintained through reflexive modes of sucking, grasping and crying. The task of the normal autistic phase is to establish homeostatic equilibrium (base line) from physiological tension. Mahler et al quotes Ribble "*As Ribble (1943) has pointed out, it is by way of mothering that the young infant is gradually brought out of an inborn tendency toward vegetative, splanchnic regression into increased sensory awareness of, contact with, the environment. [4]* In other words, through interaction with mother and the growing awareness that mother relives tension, the infant slowly becomes conscious that *relief comes from a partnership*, which the infant and mother are joined in together, the dual-unit operating as self (delusional). This dim awareness is the beginning of the *symbiosis phase* (or the dual-unit delusional phase).

Symbiosis Phase

Symbiosis in the real sense is a mutual beneficial relationship between two different organisms. Mahler's symbiosis *is a metaphor* to explain the *infant's innate perception* that he resides within the nuclear orbit with mother, and that their mutual beneficial relationship is omnipotent, from which he is the center. We now see a new and powerful (delusional and onset of narcissist perception) dual-unit of infant-mother. The autistic shift into symbiosis granted the infant upgrades! The infant now perceives mother as a powerful extension of self. Mahler explains the symbiotic relationship between mother and infant in this way "*The infant behaves and functions as though he and his mother were an omnipotent system – a dual unity within a common boundary [4].* The infant's delusional concept suggests that he is much greater and grandiose then really he is. In other words, the infant cannot conceptualize mine from not mine, and I from not-I. It is as though there is a fusion that reverberates between mother and infant. For example: The infant's feels tension and cries. The cry is routed though the symbiotic system (mother-infant dyad) from which he is the center, and the tension is relieved by his 'wish' (mother is an extension of himself) and this validates, was it called, his *primary narcissism (Ferencizi's stage of absolute or unconditional hallucinatory omnipotence." [4]).* Narcissism is facilitated though the delusion that mother is an extension of self, which of course would appear that his is greater and more powerful then he really is. However, during the symbiosis stage, primary narcissism (healthy) is a phenomenon that helps relive the infant of anxiety until he has the psychological structures to activate more sophisticated defense mechanisms. In the meantime, the dual unit of infant-mother would be much like an analogy of a dream in which one 'wishes' the pencil to rise, and magically, it rises.

(Note: it is this nexuses dream like state, this blissful belief of tranquility that imprints a powerful "symbiotic libidinal pull" (SLP) in the newly formed structures within the infant's pathology. Gradually this pathology is repressed into the unconscious, but remains a force, a regressive pull to return to oneness-with-mother, a libidinal (a libidinal - force of love, a pull to be one-with-creation).

Separation – Individuation

Separation - individuation *consists of four subphases* that begin about 4 to 5 months through 30 to 36 months. During this complex phase the infant 'hatches' out of the symbiotic orbit of the mother-infant dyad. This is achieved through progressions and regressions, frustrations and satisfactions, conflicts and resolutions between the infant and the "good-enough" (Winnicott) mother. In other words, until now, the infant's primitive cogitation and limited experiences allowed the infant to reside within the all-nurturing membrane. However, though the accumulation of experiences and the increasing sophistication of internal structures (cogitation), the membrane can on longer contain the infant, and the infant 'hatches' out into the world of separation individualization.

Separation – Individuation four subphases

(1) Differentiation

Onset at 4 to 5 months. In the *holding environment* (Winicott) of mother's arms, the infant softly becomes aware of self. This is observed when the infant stiffens and pushes away from mother as if to see mother (as other) and the environment from a different perspective. This is the launch of the distancing process with the increasing awareness of his autonomy. Mahler et al states "*As soon as the infant's apparatuses mature sufficiently, he may slide down from mother's lap, thence he crawls, paddles, and sill later walks away from mother*" [4].

(2) Practicing 10-12 / 16-18

At this point there is a shift into the beginning of a partnership between the infant being secure in the remnants of the symbiotic orbit with mother AND the infant practicing exploration into his exciting new world. It is a marvelous combination! It is as though the toddler projects a magnificent aural of "I am invincible! (Primary narcissism is at its peak!) Not only do I have these new autonomy skills and the onset of upright locomotion (like the teen that gets a new set of wheels) but I also have mother's essence to keep me safe!" Mahler points out that "*During the practicing subphase mother continues to be needed as a stable point – a "home base" to fulfill the need for refueling through physical contact. We see seven to ten-month-olds crawling or rapidly paddling to mother, righting themselves on her leg. The phenomenon was termed by Furer "emotional refueling."*

As practicing subphase evolves, the toddler gets caught up in the excitement of his investigations and discoveries. This distraction gives the impression that he is more resistant to frustration. For example, if a toy is taken away, no problem, there is a huge reservoir of other adventures waiting. In addition, the toddler is not as concerned with mother's whereabouts for longer durations of time. But of course, as in our analogy with the teen, any new set of wheels requires fuel from time to time. The toddler, like the teen, will "emotionally refuel" by tagging home base (mother) until his reservoirs are temporally replenished for another excursion. For now, the toddler is much to busy to realize that his physical distancing from mother is also creating an emotional separation from her as well. In other words, the symbiotic orbit is losing ground to his cognitive awareness that the delusional dual unit of 'we' does not exist, but rather a "me" and "not me." Yet for now, the toddler is much like a pendulum with the upswing into the clouds, that is, until the accumulation of gravity (reality) forces the pendulum into a different direction.

(3) Rapprochement (16-18 / 22-24 months)

This is perhaps the most critical stage of the separation individuation process. Settlage states "*The relative lack of separation anxiety and obliviousness to the mother's presence characteristic of the practicing phase is, in the rapprochement phase, replaced by an acutely heightened separation anxiety and active approaches to the mother, along with a seemingly constant concern with her whereabouts. [2]* The toddler is becoming acutely aware of his separation from mother; compared to his early delusion that mother was an omnipotent extension of himself. As the symbiotic safety net diminishes, his separation anxiety gains momentum. The toddler is more concerned with mother's whereabouts and demonstrates his anxiety through *active approach behavior* (rapprochement). To make things for difficult for the toddler, he is not able avail himself as easily to his 'contact supplies' in mother as he was in the past. There is a mutual realization between mother and toddler that he can do more and more for himself. Consequently, mother's response to the toddler's anxiety and frustrations are at greater and greater intervals, and *the toddler's defense to this crisis is an active approach.* We call this rapprochement.

Separation is more pronounced due to the onset of verbal progress. Separation becomes further apparent due to nouns "mine" and "me" and especially 'no.' Of course the pervasive and intrinsic component of 'no' is '*my way and not your way*, which establishes a continual awareness 'self' that is splitting away from the symbiotic orbit of 'us', the dual unit. In other words, repetition of "no" is a way of practicing the individuality of "I am." What seems negativistic may actually be positive process toward developmental growth.

Often theorists suggest that rapprochement is specifically vulnerable in the separation individualization sequence because of possible unaligned growth spurts. For example, if the toddler's gains access (growth spurt) to his upright locomotion (individualization through new experiences) before he is developmentally ready to emotionally separate from mother (separation) then the toddler is at risk for overwhelming anxiety. Because mother is not as available to metabolize and modulate the toddler's intolerable affect (mood, feelings), he is subject to the perils of abnormal pathology. This observation suggests that is helpful and a benefit to the toddler when individualization is aligned with separation from mother. A considerable acceleration or lag in either environment can manifest as disturbances throughout the life cycle.

(4) Object Constancy

As the child ushers into this phase of object constancy, his intervals through the rapprochement crises began to wax and wane. Through the repeated comings and goings of mother (establishing consistency), AND through the toddler's genetic ability to adapt (ego endowment), a new image begins to shape internally. The toddler's capacity to internalize mother through memory traces serves as a source of comfort and security when she is not available. The essence of the nurturing and soothing mother is gaining ground and is *internalized as a constant object*. We call this *object constancy.*

New tools are quickly becoming available to aid the senior toddler to cope with anxiety. His verbal communication skills are rapidly expanding. He has a growing sense of time and the meaning of "now" and "later" to aid with frustration delay. Time is not as narrowed or pressured through the relief of the internalized constant object.

III. In Depth on Rapprochement Behaviors and Complexes

Shadowing and Darting Away.

This dynamic operates like a push-pull behavior. In essence, the child runs away from mother and expects to be swooped up in the safety of her arms. Ambivalence is striking and evident since the child wishes for dependence on mother (shadowing) and then independence (darting away). It becomes a flirtatious game of play, of testing new capacities toward independence. It can also become an ambivalent nightmare. However, there are times the junior toddler may not wish to be swooped up and may react with rage on contact. Other times the child is permitted greater expansions that may lead to the engulfment of the void, and this emptiness may also cause rage. To the observer it appears as a no-win situation. During this period the child is in an emotional crises and cannot tolerate ambivalence.

Abandonment

When a child becomes separated from mother before he is emotionally ready, his libido reserves may not be sufficiently in place to overcome separation anxiety. This anxiety engenders insecurity and neediness.

The rapprochement toddler is peculiarly vulnerable due to his increasing autonomy along with his elevated cognation. He can no longer contain the illusion of the symbiotic orbit that he and mother operate as one. As the rapprochement toddler separates, his individualization is more apparent because reality is gaining ground. There is a growing realization that mother will not share in his quest for new discoveries at his beck-and-call. We now have a clash. The elated 'superman' qualities from the practicing phase (NPD) are now head-on with the depressive and anxiety rapprochement phase (BPD). The toddler has gone from a 'high' to a 'low' in a short time during the shift from one phase to the next. Some theorists speculate that resolution of the rapprochement phase sets toddler's 'base mood' for life. This model suggests that is it prudent that good-enough mother establishes attunement with her toddler to survive the rapprochement crisis.

A child that is deprived from being emotionally refueled can be haunted with pervasive emptiness and a lack of identify, or a loss of self. This is how one fixated adult put it:

It's hard to be a child in a grown up world. It's a feeling of being lost. It's sad sometimes because when I see other children they don't look lost. They have parents, structure and guidelines. This helped them grow and form into an adult. They went through the maze and arrived at the other end. It was a maze I have never had the opportunity to enter. What is structure? I remember at 6 being on the other side of town in the blackness of the night. No one cared where I was. What are parents? I can't ever remember being loved, rocked, cuddled or held. I have no memory traces of this. What are guidelines? I had none and made them up as I went along in life. I'm afraid my guidelines are not very stable since I didn't have a measuring stick that was constant in my life. Is it any wonder that I am still a lost child that is pretending to be an adult?

Engulfment

On the flip side, a mother that projects her insecurities (i.e. obsession with perfection, fear) onto her infant through constant handling can prevent the infant's satisfaction through exploration. With mother's incessant patterns of containment, the infant may resent her encroachment of his expanding world. The infant may learn to scan the restricted environment for opportunities to experience his independence. As the child progresses, engulfment may looked as though it were a glass bubble. Freedom is imposed and deferred to inappropriate responsibilities that gives the impression the child is a 'little adult.' This encroaches on his developing identity since to 'mother himself' takes on a distorted view of individually in the formation of the false-self. In other words, the child is being taken intellectually advantage of with no regard for his developmental and emotional lag. Kramer validates "Cut off from the needed relationship and parental regulatory help, the child is at the mercy of the inner impulses and feelings...the child does not experience the usual parental pleasure in the child's growth. Instead, the child feels used in the service of the parent's anxieties and needs [1]. In a clear sense, this can be seen when the older child assumes the adult role of caretaker without sufficient provision for libidinous nurturing and affection. A child that is saddled with added responsibilities without appropriate developmental nurturing is at risk for developmental fixation.

The Rapprochement Crisis

As the child becomes psychically and cognitively aware of his new budding world, he becomes increasingly conscious that he can no longer maintain his delusional symbiotic orbit with mother. Mahler states that *"While individuation proceeds very rapidly and the child exercises it to the limit, he also becomes more and more aware of his separateness from mother."* The crisis of the rapprochement subphase heightens as the child realizes mother is not an extension of himself, but he is rather a small, helpless diminutive individual.

In contrast to the practicing phase when the child's narcissism was at its peak and the world was his oyster sort of speak, the child is now overwhelmed with narcissist injury on a daily basis. The world that seemed as a treasure trove for new opportunities to conquer with his new ambulatory locomotion during the practicing phase is now being delineated by the harsher psychical boundaries of reality. He cannot do as he anticipated. It begins to dawn on him that he is not as grandiose or powerful as his first imagined.

Transitional Object

Winnicott who coined the term transitional object suggested that the child intimately cathected (energized) the object (diaper, blanket, etc) with the libidinal investment of mother. "*Transitional objects tend to be soft and are capable of being cuddly; they help evoke primitive memories of being held, comforted, fed and, importantly, played with. Eventually, probably 70 percent of children in separately bedded situations (Ekecranz and Ruhde 1971) have transitional objects (blankets, diapers, stuffed animals)[8]*. The cathexis of the transitional object usually begins during the preverbal period and depending on the resolution of the separation - individualization phase, the transitional object may take on a more pervasive function to ease anxiety. It is important to note that the transitional object is within the complete control of the child and yielding unlike the individually of mother. This serves the purpose to help the child separate from mother because the transitional object is available when needed or can be discarded during periods of exploration.

Once the child displays his limited independent abilities, his mother may resent or refuse to partake in his regressive dependencies and the child may feel emotionally abandoned. Other times the when child may be libidinally (love, nurturing, essence) separated from mother via a phone call, or more physically, out of the room for long periods of time. Since the child's increasing awareness of separation embarks on the transitional period, the transitional object takes on a greater significance if mother is not emotionally available to supply the child with object libido. To help ease libidinal separations the child cathexed an object with representation of mother. Bergman summarizes "*The transitional object (Winnicott 1953) of the early months is a object found by the baby which stands between the self- and the object world and provides a safe intermediary area of experience which allows both separateness and fusion.*" [2]

Resolution vs. Progression of the Transitional Object

As the child progress through the separation-individualization stages, there is a shift toward object constancy. Maternal supplies bridged with the transitional object can help a child to *transition* from the powerful influence of the infant-mother dyadic position (symbiotic dual unit), to the *"first meaningful triangulation of the infant-mother dyad, the transitional object [8]."* The temporary transitional object (aid/support –temporary maternal supply) paves the way to a consistent internalized representation of maternal nurturing and soothing (object constancy) when mother is not available. Grolnick explains, *"Transitional objects and phenomena are only the first steps toward the development of, hopefully, an equally treasured symbolic and cultural world."* [8]

Disturbance in the Transitional Period

Yet on occasion because of the child's genetic endowment and inability to internalize the maternal object into a satisfactory holding environment, the transitional object remains. It is not uncommon for an individual to puzzle over the idea what went wrong? They may reason, "I had a great childhood and etc." However, since developmental phases are largely repressed and unconscious, preverbal disturbances are elusive. Perhaps through professional deconstruction, confrontation, examination and the realignment genetic endowment, the unconscious may be brought into the conscious. What may appear as a 'normal' rapprochement crisis for one child may completely, and chronically overwhelm another child to create an almost psychotic cathected transitional object. In other words, there is a fixation of libido energy during the transitional period that did not get recathected. To hold and resonate with the transitional object, is to hold and resonate with maternal handling. What remains is the artifact, the libidinally cathected transitional object. Bergman suggests, *"It would seem that that the transitional object serves the illusion of oneness…"* [2]

IV. Separation Individuation Disturbances

The failure to reach a resolution during the developmental phase can have far reaching implications. "As old, partially unresolved sense of self-identity and of body boundaries, or old conflicts over separation and separateness, can be reactivated (or remain peripherally or even centrally active) at any and all stages of life…"

Autism

Mahler suggests that in <u>some</u> cases the infant will not hatch out of his autistic orbit if an attunement with mother is too painful. In other words, the infant retreats into his own internal world. The communication between mother and infant are out of sync. The task to resolve the miscommunication may frustrate and prevent the joint path into the symbolic dual unit. The miscommunication may be grounded in the infant's ego endowment and advancement is too painful, therefore the infant retreats into the autistic realm where mother's smile is not mirrored back to her.

Symbiotic Libidinal Pull (SLP)

Matterson found that treating certain patients was difficult because there "*is still a strong internal regressive pull to maintain the old familiar rewarding object relations unit*" [11]. The Symbiotic Libidinal Pull (SLP) derives from the unconscious attraction to the symbiotic orbit of the mother-infant dyad that was experienced when mother was conceptualize as an extension of the self (symbiotic phase), as a container that resolved and metabolized anxiety through her affect modulation. The strength of the SLP is a regressive force, an energy, a 'pull". SLP is conceptualized as a nexuses, a oneness with creation, a completeness. For example, this force to return, to regress is exemplified with the rival of baby into the family unit in the face of an older child.

> Here we see "*another form of attempted adaptation was identification with the rival baby. Matthew showed signs of wanting to be a baby himself; like this baby brother, of instance, he would climb into the playpen* [4]. Mother was intolerant of his regressive behavior and Matthew; the happy radiant child began to adapt aggressive conduct by throwing objects out of frustration. It was observed that Matthew had lost his spark for life in service of the mother, the influence of the false-self, "*all of which on superficial observation seemed to be in compliance with mother's wishes that he be independent and remain her happy little "big" boy* [4].

The influence of the SLP will vary depending on the progress on the separation - individualization phase. The greater the symbolic pull, the more likely the individual is developmentally conflicted with unsatisfactory object constancy. If the individual's development is static and held in abeyance because insufficient maternal reserves are absent or not fully integrated, the individual may become fixated and employ primitive defensive mechanisms (regressions, splitting and etc.) to relieve anxiety.

SLP, Anxiety and Defense Mechanisms

To simplify, anxiety derives from three sources (pressures) of conflict. To simplify, they are (1) pleasure seeking (impulsive) and the aspects needed to survive, (2) morals and perfection, formed out of punishment and rewards, and (3) the external world (reality). Depending on the source of conflict, defense mechanisms are automatically activated to prevent the individual from the harshness of reality. Defense mechanisms distort or distract an individual from the full impact of reality. If the defense mechanism(s) is successful, a compromise has been reached between the opposing forces toward a decision that enables the discharge or displacement of anxiety. However, when defensives are primitive or ridged, and the personality is rendered with inflexibility, then there is likely a disturbance in the Separation - Individualization phase that is yielding to the SLP. In other words, the inability to defuse anxiety renders the individual prey to the regressive, symbiotic magnetic pull of oneness with creation. Primitive defenses closely orbit the SLP due to its greater gravitational pull, then the more distant orbits of sophisticated defenses.

Brief Discussion on Defense Mechanisms.

At birth, the infant has no need for defense mechanisms because the ego has not evolved out of the autistic orbit into an awareness that requires a defense. Defense mechanisms protect the ego (self) from anxiety by distorting reality. Defense mechanisms are largely unconscious. Lets run through several of them.

Primitive Defenses (Close orbit to the SLP)

Regression: Return to an earlier developmental level of functioning prompt by anxiety. For example, an individual overtaken with losses collapsed into a fetal position. An adult clutches a stuffed bunny (transitional object) to ease anxiety. A child temporarily reverts to dependence as a relief from the new responsibilities of independence.

Splitting: Separation of internal objects that create anxiety. For example individuals that cannot tolerate ambivalence (shades of gray) will split a person as 'all-good' or 'all-bad.' It creates less anxiety to completely hate a person that is 'all bad.'

Projection: Decrease anxiety by deferring responsibility onto others. It is easier to tolerate 'You made me do it' rather then 'I did it."

Projection Identification: Projection with intense pressure. There is a decrease in anxiety when pushing an individual into a role to preserve perception. Altering perception would create a mass upheaval within the mind. It is easier to tolerate "He is a liar" by massive projection. This defense creates a target to deposit the hate that resides within the self. In other words, "If I treat you like the bad object long enough, you will become the bad object, and then I have a 'right' to hate you." We could say the treater became the bad object through projective identification.

Denial: Stops anxiety dead in its tracks. "How can I be upset if it didn't happen?"

Sophisticated Defenses (Distant orbit to the SLP)

Rationalization: Excusing the behavior through an internal debate. "So what? I would have happened sooner or later anyway." Rationalization defends against internalized moral and cultural conflicts.

Intellectualization: The use of abstract thought to advert or minimize troublesome emotions (anxiety). For example, a man avoids the emotional grief from the loss of his wife by intellectualizing she had a long life in spite of her illness.

Repression: Evading unwanted anxiety through avoidance. Usually repression is the source from which other defense mechanisms operate. For example the repression of early trauma protects the psych from anxiety.

Sublimation: The release of anxiety through more appropriate and 'acceptable' channels. For example, an individual may release his rage in a sport such as boxing.

Reaction Formation: Behaving the complete opposite of one's true desires to avoid anxiety. For example, a pedophile becomes a priest to advert unacceptable impulses. An employee is extra nice to her boss whom she hates to save her job.

Identification: Identification with a role model, parent, teacher etc to avoid anxiety within the self. For example, identification with a committee, a wining team, or organization can deflect anxiety through absorption and participation.

Maturity vs. Fixation and Object Constancy

After separation – individualization has been sufficiently resolved; a more mature defense against the SLP has evolved. The child is able to internalize a consistent, available image and the essence of mother though repeated satisfactory (good enough) interactions with her. The child's integrated conceptualization of mother satisfies the demands of the SLP and helps regulate anxiety. We call this object constancy.

As the child matures and the SLP is adequately satisfied with the constant internalized mother object, a new dynamic begins to take shape reaching into youth and adulthood. The constant object within the youth/adult reverberates with the SLP to form a more integrated sense of self, a new dual unit. The self becomes integrated within the self, no longer seeking the maternal nurturing though the original symbolic mother - infant dyad. What has emerged is an individual that has separated from the unconscious nexuses of mother. The individual is now ready to enter into a more mature libidinous relationship with 'other', a life partner.

In the absence of the more mature (integrated) sense of self due to disturbance in the separation individualization phase, manifestations to recreate and replay a failed situation in hopes of a better outcome can become chronically and compulsively intrinsic with the individual's pathology. Treaters find this especially difficulty according to Matterson and Chathan *"They bring nothing into the treatment that will disrupt the symbiotic fantasized relationship with the therapist and thus activate depression [11].*

V. Symbiotic Libidinal Pull (SLP) and Manifestations

Because SLP is a regressive force, its vicissitudes may become apparent though the manifestation of unusual behaviors. These behaviors are the result of mechanisms that were created to satisfy the unconscious demands for emotional equilibrium.

Transitional Object Revisited

The transitional object is a defense against the demands of the SLP. The cathected object may enable functioning and impede regression. The transitional object represents a compromise for the unconscious need of maternal supply. In this vignette temporary relief was intermediately attained though contact with the transitional object. An example:

> *A forty-year-old patient reported that in times of anxiety or insecurity her 'center' would 'pull.' At times the patient would appear crunched over with her hands pressing on her stomach to hold her 'insides in' because the pull was so pervasive. To access relief she would carry a transitional object to establish emotional equilibrium (homeostasis). This worked quite well for her most of the time. Other times her transitional object failed when her 'center' pulled with an enormous tension. At those times she would regress and not be able to function.*

In preceding vignette the transitional object was the first line of defense against regression. Another example of a transitional object is medication. The patient emotionally refueled when taking her pills that represented the nurturing care of her idealized doctor. Perhaps the placebo effect can be explained in the transitional phenomena. In other words, the (fake) pill worked because it was cathected as transitional object.
We can also see the comforting influence of the transitional object in this case:

> *"Blanck and Blanck (1979,pp. 156-157) have discussed the use of the transitional objects when the therapist cannot meet with the patients. For example, when they went on vacation, they have one severely disturbed woman their phone number on a piece of paper so that she could have it as a transitional object. The woman never telephoned them, but she felt secure just having the number [11].*

The author makes the point clear that the transitional object can help maintain the object image of the treater to soothe anxiety.

Transvestite Manifestation

Disturbance during the rapprochement crisis though sudden, unexpected and prolonged separations with mother can affect the structure building process of the internalized *constant object* representing mother (The forth subphase). Because there is a disturbance with the libidinous internalized representation of mother, the symbiotic libidinal pull (SLP) manifests in child's behavior in an unconscious attempt to preserve the relationship. In this example the child does not understand 'why' he behaves the why he does, only that it satisfies the demand of the SLP through manifestation of symbiotic representation.

Settlage Case [1]

> A 3-year-old boy became preoccupied with girlish activities and insisted on dressing up in mother's clothes, wearing her jewelry, putting on her perfume and cosmetics, and carrying a purse. At the same time, he showed little or no interest in boyish activities and pursuits.
>
> Beginning at age 18 months, the boy experienced repeated disruptions of his relationship with his mother. She reported that she felt compelled to leave the house. Having made arrangements for a caregiver, she did so, sometimes several times a day. His attempting to become like or identical with mother severed to nullify the threat of separation.

Here we see the genesis pathology in transvestitism. I suggest that transvestitism occurs more often in the male gender because it is mother who gave birth and the separation individualization process is more difficult based on alignment of gender identity differences and the cultural demands on males (big boys don't cry, etc…).

Infantilism Manifestation

In <u>*true infantilism*</u> the individual's pathology is centered on the transitional object. Depending upon the strength of the SLP from disturbances in the separation individualization phase, an individual may have a neurotic compulsion to regress because the individual is seeking a component of maternal satisfaction from the cathected transitional object rather then in 'other.' Usually in infantilism there is object fragmentation (splitting) and the internalized representation of the maternal object is not integrated into a continuing sense of self. During these times 'significant other' is not seen as a whole cohesive individual to in their own right, but rather as maternal supply for fusion to satisfy the primitive symbiotic orbit of oneness with creation – mother.

In relationships, coping with fragmentation may be problematic since the fragmented individual oscillates between the need to emotionally refuel with maternal supplies (symbiotic orbit) AND the need to express intimacy in age appropriate manner. The spouse however, is usually an integrated individual that has developmentally matured and cannot understand the significance of the transitional object. For example the significant other may reason, "I should be able to libidinally satisfy all your needs. Toss the transitional object." However, because the individual is fragmented, and the split-off infantile object (part-self) is developmentally fixated, the resonating transitional object and its concomitants remain as a source for maternal supplies. It is almost as though there is a dual personality (fragmented) in which the individual seeks 'balance.'

Reparenting

This is a difficult decision and can open up a can of worms. Reparenting if not done correctly can come off as a reintroduction to the SLP abyss. The formation of a malignant regression can be dangerous when it shifts into a realm of impossibility. However, a benign regression can be most helpful and therapeutic.

The benign regressions are carried out as goals focused through excises to progress through developmental fixation. For example, a patient is regressed when old unresolved hurts (transferences / distortions) resurface and are directed toward the treater. For the more fragmented individual, integration takes place through the taking in of (introjection) positive interactions with the treater. Lets say old wounds are resurrected, amplified (unresolved rage) and projected onto the treater, (the treater is the target of transferences), it is the treater's function to empathetically acknowledged the rage (projected object in the transference), and handle resurrected dynamics of the rage by taking it in, detoxifying the rage, and offer it back in a less threatening form. In other words, the patients close core structures are modified when the treater acknowledges the rage first, and then helps defuse the situation as a new role model (identification). For example the regressed patient may say, "I HATE you! You are just like my mother! You always twist things around!" The treater responds, "I can see you are angry, really mad. I would be mad too if my mother twisted everything around. I bet being misunderstood would be crazy making. So if things appear as twisted around, lets figure out what happened because I wouldn't be doing my part to let you go on thinking that." Here we see the treater has accepted the rage, contained it, and is now aligning a positive and corrective stance with the patient, (the patient has split off the bad object in the transference, projected into the treater, and the treater as contained, detoxified the bad object, now modified, and offered it back in a

more harmless form to the patient). What the treater has done in effect, has reparented the patient and built a stronger trust, with means, *strengthen the therapeutic alliance.* Once this alliance has become stronger, and the bad objects in the patient has been modified through repeated interactions with the treater, which after a time, will bring us to the next step.
Be forewarned, this usually works only for the more integrated individual. Through clarification, confrontation and interpretation, the regression in transference promotes growth through insight and self-awareness and especially through the cathartic release, (great pain released in tears).

The malignant and dangerous regressions into reparenting would be the sinking of self, fused with the powerful SLP. Rule of thumb, regressions are benign and helpful when they promote growth to a period of moving on. Regressions are malignant when they become the object of fusion and static with the symbiotic magnetic pull, and there is no relief, but more of a demand for unreasonable entitlement. The task of reparenting should take place in the framework of structured holding environment because it can act as the safety net from the abyss of the SLP.

Borderline Personality Manifestation

The hallmark traits of borderline personality disorder (BPD) are a lack of identity, pervasive emptiness, excessive anger and the inability to regulate emotion. The sources of these symptoms were caused by the dynamic, ambivalent and powerful struggle between the SLP vs. individualization during the rapprochement subphase. *"The rapprochement subphase is where the fixation becomes apparent, with the point of origin in the symbiotic phase [11].* Here we see dependence vs. independence.

Emptiness – the lack of a maternal constant object

Since the subphase of object constancy has not developed within the borderline individual, he resides predominately within the rapprochement subphase. There is a constant reverberation of the push-pull behavior. A sort of "I hate you, don't leave me' or 'I run away, come rescue me' dynamic. We see this because a borderline individual has not internalized the 'all-good nurturing maternal object' (emptiness) and when his fleeting maternal supplies diminish, there is a run-away behavior to prompt the chase. We can sum it up in this way, *"If you catch me, you love me, if you don't catch me, you hate me."* When 'captured' the borderline individual's maternal supplies are replenished for a time. We can see this clearly when the borderline patient tries to woo and extract maternal attention from the treater. If the treater fails, like the toddler, the borderline patient will up-the-stakes, sort of speak. Note this observation in the toddler. *"It is quite impressive to observe the extent to which the normal infant-toddler is intent upon extracting, and in usually able to extract, contact supplies and participation from the mother, sometimes against considerable odds; how he tries to incorporate every bit of these supplies into libidinal channels for progressive personality organization [9].* Here we see that the borderline individual is behaving as the normal toddler through rapprochement with his treater. The problem a treater faces is that *active approaching* (rapprochement) and the 'catch' appears as chronic, and therefore draining on the reserves of the therapeutic relationship. Sooner or later the therapeutic relationship with the borderline individual will take the normal course into a rapprochement crisis that is age appropriate with the toddler. What may appear to a treater as 'regression' is actually a resuming course of development that was fixated in childhood.

Rage

The hallmark of the borderline individual is rage. Rage from the separation of the maternal symbiotic orbit without the compensation of the internalized maternal constant object because the resolution of the rapprochement subphase has failed. Rage derived from the repeated failure of environment's attunement with the infant's inborn ego endowment. In other words, the child has failed to get what he needs because of problems from attunement with the primary love object or from abuse. The oscillation of rage is directly in sync with the borderline's fluctuation of maternal supplies from his environment. Since a constant object does not exist within the borderline individual, then the constant modulation to defuse rage does not exist either. The containment of rage is much like the containment of maternal effect. Neither are subject to containment without external attention. To say it another way, the borderline individual is able to contain his rage as well as he is able to contain the constant object, which is to say, not very well. Note this observation. "Rage tends to wipe out positive experience in relationships and maintain a predominance of angry over loving feelings. Good experience fails to "stick to the ribs" of psychic structure" [1]. This is why in borderline individuals we see the rollercoaster affect. Their moods are fluid and can begin or end abruptly in direct relation to the success of the rapprochement catch.

Treatment

The goal of the treater is to experiment and develop an attunement with the borderline individual. Through validation and positive mirroring a strong therapeutic alliance can be constructed. One of the signs of a strong alliance is the resumption of the rapprochement subphase that will move forward into the rapprochement crisis. Here we see the flare up of rage, which seems puzzling because things were going so well as the alliance developed. We use the analogy in which rage is like nuclear fusion and if not contained can be a bomb. However, nuclear fusion can be contained in specially built nuclear power plants (holding environment) and the energy (rage) can be modified. It is important to note that without fusion (rage-heat) there is nothing to modify (structural change). The negative affects that were repressed due to failed attunement or abuse are resurrected in the holding environment. If the treater is successful, rage from the negative affects is modified into the formation of the internalized constant object.

Treaters face problems when they 'are afraid to upset the patient' and employ all sorts of tactics to maintain a positive affect in the patient. The holding environment that was constructed for fusion is not utilized. Sessions are uneventful, boring and dead. Some treaters take the low road to pass the time in chitchat. This would be much like a blacksmith attempting to shape a cold chuck of metal without heat. However, with the application of heat, and the skillful use of development tools, the blacksmith is able to modify the metal.

Working with the borderline individual is an art and similar to the navigation of a vehicle because there must be balance of acceleration and breaking to get someplace. Breaking (speed regulation in dangerous areas) is akin to the establishment and promotion of positive affects (positive transferences) to maintain the holding environment that is needed for treatment compliance. In other words, the strength of the alliance and the ability to get something done is based on the positive emotion toward the treater. Acceleration (working through – going somewhere) is the application of negative affects (negative transferences) that generate anger and rage. The treater's employment of developmental skills can reshape the psychic structures while contained within the holding environment.

However, the treater must be prudent not to pervasively overwhelm the patient with negative affect since to do so would equate to a car going over a cliff (the therapeutic alliance has severally deteriorated and cannot be repaired). During these times breaking (use of positive affects), and backing off on acceleration (shelving negative affects) can preserve the alliance. This will give the client a chance to fall back and regroup. This attunement carries the rapprochement crisis forward through regressions – progressions, unavailability – availability, and rage – soothing. It is the successful reverberation of comings and goings with the treater that produces useful derivatives in the formation of the constant object.

The Holding Environment

This term, coined by Winnicott suggested the treater create a holding space, which can provide a safe place for experimentation and change with the patient. Winnicott emphasized that the critical element of the holding environment was its framework, or operating boundaries. To help prevent unnecessary treatment failures Winnicott suggested explaining to the patient *at the onset* of treatment an agreement between the therapist and patient. For example, lateness is handled this way, or missed sessions in this way, or dangerous behaviors in this way. Be consistent! How can the patient internalize a constant object if the treater does not model one?!

Action should take place as matter-of-factly without irritation (countertransference reaction). This is especially important with personalities that are prone to feel slighted without perfect mirroring. In other words, a treater that changes the rules as he goes can have a deadly effect. It may come off as the 'rejecting mirror' and validate beliefs, and destroy months carefully constructed introjects that modified the patients poor objects relations. The treater that changes the rules as he goes may come off as a cheater, weak, passive, aggressive or a whole range of affects. And, the patient with a ridged and unforgiving personality (rightly so in many cases) will walk or act out dangerously and then, treatment has failed.

It is important to discuss with the patient the difference between 'acting out' (physical aggression, missed or late appointments, dangerous behaviors) and 'working through.' Working though is the verbalization of feelings, emotions and affect. Acting out on the other hand must confronted using a preset framework of consequences. For example, consequences (other then the execution boundary) can strengthen the therapeutic alliance. In some cases consequences will validate the rapprochement-patient that he as been 'caught' in the unconscious compulsion to 'shadow and dart away.' Much in the same way as the rapprochement-toddler, object constancy will progress for the patient through testing, the comings and goings of the treater.

Transitional Space

Once the holding environment is constructed it can provide a safe place for transition. Winnicott viewed the transitional space (the transitional phenomena) as an intermediate space to invite experimentation and exploration. It was modeled from the mother-infant transitional space during the separation-individualization phase. It is sort of a playground, a place to assign roles that are resurrected from the past (transferences) and played out. As these roles take shape, a distorted reverberation based in the past (transferences - countertransferences) will take place between the treater and the patient. For example a treater may kindle an exaggerated rage in the patient from slight rejections. In other words the joint assigned roles between the treater and the patient has stirred emotions of the over critical and rejecting parent. Once the roles are in motion in a safe place (activated transferences of the bad object in the transitional space) the treater guides the treatment course with skillful tools. The skillful treater may apply more 'heat' to ambiguous transitions to bring clarity, to help the situation become more obvious. Usually, during a return to baseline there is a *cathartic release* within the patient from repressed emotions. Guidance from the treater in the form of clarification, confrontation and interpretation can crystallize the flooding of emotions into a meaningful experience. This is similar to our analogy of the blacksmith that quenches the carefully shaped metal in the water. The modified metal is crystallized as the steam escapes, much as the patient is modified as the repressed emotions escape the cold labyrinths of confusion…. all while in Winnicott's transitional space within the framework of the holding environment.

Narcissist Personality Manifestation

Unlike the borderline individual fixated in the rapprochement subphase, the narcissist individual is fixated in the earlier practicing subphase. Narcissistic manifestation originates from the infant's inability to separate from the grandiose delusional derivatives of the symbiotic orbit. This poses as a curiosity (Masterson) because the infant 'develops' through the rapprochement crisis consisting of successes and failures. I say curious because in order for the infant to separate from mother, the infant would have to had actually experienced the successful resolution of environmental difficulties based in reality, and of course since the resolutions are reality based, one would expect the infant to have realized through such experiences that he is NOT as powerful or grandiose as he perceived he was at the height of the practicing phase. In other words, the dilemma can be postulated in this analogy "How does an individual acquire financial credit, if the individual does not have the required credit history?" For instance a banker may say, "I'm sorry, you do not have a credit history. We cannot give you the money." The response is, "How can I get a credit history if I cannot get a loan to began with?!" Of course to circumvent the banker's requirement, the individual can provide phony credit documents. Basically, that is to lie. So, we now see the infant was manipulated to lie (use defense mechanisms [denial et al] to 'bypass' the rapprochement crisis.)

Back to our narcissistic model, the infant distorts (lies) on an unconscious level though the primitive defenses of denial, projection and splitting to maintain the illusion that he is STILL powerful and grandiose. But why would the infant feel pressured into distorting though denial?

Lets say mother is projecting her needs and insecurities into the infant. The infant feels obligated to engage and to expend his energy to satisfy mother else he may risk losing her love. In the infant's engagement to satisfy mother, his development is arrested as he constructs psychological structures to please her needs. The infant's psychological structures shaped from the projection of mother's needs are called the false self. One of the major components of this model of the false self is the grandiose and omnipotence distortions. In other words the infant is busy clinging onto his delusion of power, because without it he would not be able to meet mothers needs, and lets face it, how many of us would lie, cheat and steal to save the life of a loved one? The infant is busy clinging onto his distortions (lying) because without them he would be small, helpless, and powerless to save mother and himself. Hence we see the infant's chronic adaptation of denial (one of many) as a defense to survive and maintain mother's love.

In this model the infant was not able to relinquish the narcissistic component so he could save mother, and therefore he could not fully benefit from the rapprochement crisis. Most of the infant's successes and failures during the rapprochement crisis were grounded in distortions (lies) and now, the result is the end product of the false self. In service of the mother, the infant gave up himself. In the military, when an individual gives up himself for his country, he is considered a hero and decorated with honors and metals. However, in contrast to the military hero, the narcissistic infant is unfairly despised for his sacrifice of self later in life.

The narcissist adult is in a very sad place. One prominent narcissistic individual (Vaknin) said, "I HATE it when a women tells me that she loves me!" On the surface this would appear confusing since love is to be desired. However, with the narcissist, love equates to obligation (mother-infant dyad), which equates to psychological death. On the unconscious level, the narcissist must HATE love in order to survive, in order to have the HOPE of finding the true self. Love to the narcissist is a force that discarded the true self into a coffin and buried it alive. Love is not to breath, but to suffocate. To reverberate with love means to throw oneself away. Of instance, the woman says, "I'm falling in love with you" translates to the narcissist on an unconscious level to "I'm beginning to obsess with the idea of murdering you."

Treatment

Treating the narcissist patient is challenging. Because the narcissist patient's development was subphase arrested, the treater must construct an environment in which to promote and encourage developmental growth. Growth for the patient occurs in the resumption of *empathy based mirroring* and/or safely idealizing the treater (mirror and/or idealizing transferences). Lets look at each of these transferences:

Mirroring - To get past the argument of defense mechanisms, conflicts and etc, Kohut looked at the 'self' as the essence, the core personality. Working with the concept of the 'total-self' enabled the role of the treater to provide mirroring and empathy that was transcendent of resistant barriers in the patient. We could say that since the narcissist personality is subphase fixated, it is therefore fragmented.

Attention is focused toward perfect mirroring, a *system of reverie* (mother validating the infant's true-self) that failed in the original developmental practicing subphase. What we are talking about is this: the patient will act-out old wounds from the past, (I will prove to you I am worthy - invalidated infant), amplify those wounds toward the treater, (I will impress you with my worthiness - invalidated infant is now the amplified invalidated adult). The treaters role is to take the, "*empathic-introspective stand, which allows him or her to be responsive to the patient's total-*

self" [11]. We see though the technique of perfect mirroring; a gradual consistently is taking place.

However, what is perfect mirroring? The narcissist will be the first to argue there is no such thing as perfection when it comes to mirroring. They should know. As infants they have unconsciously strived over and over again to win mother over though the development of the false-self as an attempt to perfectly mirror mother! And, nothing work! Interesting, for the narcissist adult to acknowledge the perfect mirror would equate to acknowledging the destruction of the self. In other words, to face perfection would be to face destruction. Because quite frankly, the narcissist has already PROVED that as infants, the perfect mirror destroyed them. It was a double loss. (1) The true self was lost at the formation of the false-self in service of the mother, and (2) Mother was also lost in the process.

What the treater can hope to achieve is dialectal mirroring. In other words, through the process of working through, the treater is able to dialectally reverie with the patient toward a common ground. In other words, the not-good-enough mirroring becomes good-enough built on sincerity, empathy, and constancy *toward a vector of perfection*. Dialectal because the patient is in need of perfect mirroring, and the treater mirrors imperfectly. The process repeats (dialectally) again, except this time a synthesis has occurred and the treater is positioned closer to the patient's unconscious appeal for perfect mirroring. So as you can see, the narcissist patient is unconsciously fragmented (splitting) into perfect mirroring vs. failed mirroring. However, through the dialectal empathic mirror, integration may be able to take place.

VI. Conclusion

We have learned that objectifying the psych into object relations can provide powerful tools to deconstruct (reverse engineer) the end product of pathology that originated in childhood. In other words, the end product of present day behaviors (i.e. neurotic, ridged, obsessive, object attachment or failure to attach) that originated in childhood can be reexamined and identified to provide insight into that which was unknown (unconscious). We have learned that fixation or arrest in a critical phase(s) during the first three years of life can have lasting implications. In some cases we have learned that 'knowing' and 'insight' is at times not enough. Treatment is necessary when a disturbed individual's quality of life is severely undermined by their pathology. *"The process of structural change involves the undoing of pathology and the resumption of development." [1]* Sometimes relief can only come from working-through with a skilled professional that has a solid foundation in developmental knowledge. There are times the professional can assist with *validation (a supportive stance of benign behaviors that provide relief)*, or a system of *working through.* Working through tackles developmental obstacles with a balance of treatment stances. Some stances are educational, supportive, confronting, or a delicate mixture of complex stances that lead (they own it) the patient to self-discovery. A treater must know when to guide, when to carry, when to support and when to intermittently let go.

We have learned about defense mechanisms. The closer their orbit to the symbiotic magnetic pull, the more primitive they are.

We have learned that change is intrinsic of the life cycle, either through re-validation (i.e. strengthen self-esteem or strengthen "I am bad") or modification (a corrective, harmful, or educative experience). We have seen how disturbances in the rapprochement subphase manifests into borderline personality organization or fixation in the practicing subphase can manifest into narcissist personality organization. Depending on the period of arrestment, developmental manifestations are *amplified at the point of fixation.* In other words, the infant will to proceed at the drop-off-point, much like a seed that fell out of the planter's pouch. Rather then grow at the planter's destination in rich soil; the seed took root where it fell. Perhaps the soil was bare (abandonment), or perhaps it was saturated (engulfment). The end result may be a stunted or distorted tree. However, the knowledgeable nurturing caretaker (treater) can prune the limbs to encourage redirection and enrich the ground with the necessary ingredients to correct and promote growth.

Test Yourself:

1. What are the two fore runners of the Separation - Individuation phase?
2. What is the dual unit of the mother - infant termed?
3. What would a security blanket for an adult or child be called?
4. What does Rapprochement mean?
5. What does Reaction Formation mean?
6. What protects the ego from anxiety (self)?
7. What term did Winnicott coin to describe the framework for treatment?
8. Which subphase may determine mood baseline for life?
9. What is the SLP?
10. What do we mean by "object?" as in object relations?
11. What are we talking about when we say, "Nature vs. Nurture?"

Breaking Free From Co-dependence

Written by Kathi Stringer

July 12, 2003

Co-dependency is a style of relating to others that could be in the form of aggression, submissiveness, people-pleaser, neediness and etc.

First, We Identify Co-dependency.

The fit. It would seem that if we put a people-pleaser with a needy person, we would have an ideal fit. We don't. What we have is co-dependence. Each person 'needs' the other person to feel 'whole' due to his or her unconscious pathology. Neither is whole in their own right but is dependent on the other to maintain a certain 'completeness.' Eventually, when each person is out-of-sync with the "giving and getting," there are accusatory problems and blame, i.e..."You don't appreciate me enough when I..." or "You never give me enough when I..." The people-pleaser cannot please enough or the needy person cannot get enough. This becomes a problem when one individual is sick of the co-dependent relationship and having to deal with the burden of being out-of-sync. What may happen next is the threat of change. This change of course does not go over well with the other individual. There is massive resistance. Why? Because change is seen in the other individual as REJECTION (a LOSS). When the people-pleaser changes, the needy person views this as REJECTION and will try and prevent this loss through all sorts of road-blocking behaviors. On the other hand, if the needy person becomes more independent, the people-pleaser is also afraid of rejection and won't be 'needed' any more. The core of both pathologies is 'rejection.'

Now, We Identify Wellness

Wholeness. When both individuals are complete in their own right, then, we have a mutual beneficial relationship. Here, each individual brings something into the 'relationship' to promote growth, rather then to patch a defect. When each individual is complete, the relationship builds and moves along. On the flip side, when individuals are 'fused' due to incompleteness, there is no movement, only a constant state of repair.

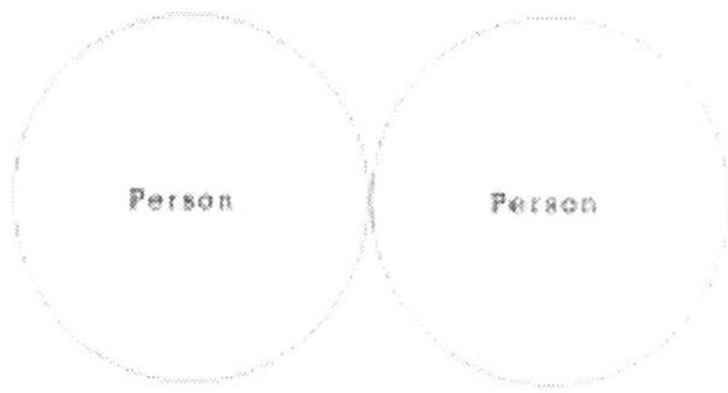

Wholeness - Wellness

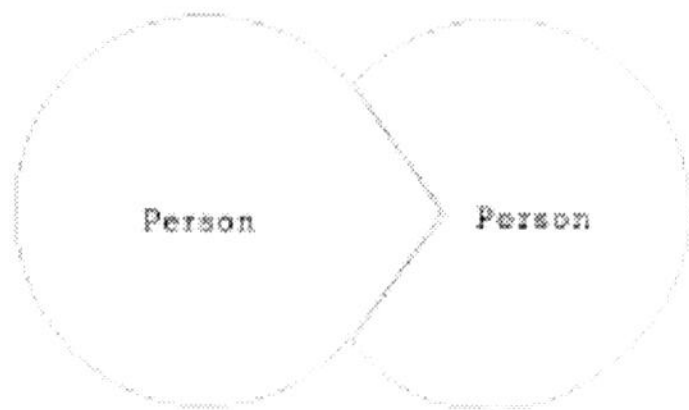

Co-dependence / FUSION

Concept and Drawing by Kathi Stringer

An analogy

Co-dependency would be like a medic on the battlefield attending to the patient. The patient is chronic and the medic will not give up. The medic continues to repair the patient over and over again. Neither of them is moving anywhere. They are stuck on the battlefield. The patient is too hurt to move and the medic is too busy repairing the patient to move himself. The patient has a false sense of security of being chronically repaired by the medic. The medic has a false sense of security of being needed by the never-healing chronic patient. On the other hand, if both were whole individuals in their own right, there would be no need for a patient or a medic. Rather, the individuals can actually meet and move on through life's journey without the cumbersome repetitiveness of chronic repair.

Solution

Change. "Nothing changes if nothing changes." Because co-dependency is FUSION, there is a major problem with change. Change in either person is seen as REJECTION to the other person. 1. If I ask and you don't give = rejection. 2. If I give and you don't take = rejection. Let's see this dynamic in motion. The people-pleaser of the family can never do enough. The takers hound the people-pleaser with criticism. The people-pleaser will ALWAYS be one short of the stack and will continue to be abused while chasing the proverbial carrot to be 'worthy of love.' The people-pleaser will break down in tears because they can never do enough or give enough. The people-pleaser is locked into a false illusion that if they finally jump high enough, run fast enough or anticipate every need well in advance, that they will finally be worthy of love. NOT A CHANCE! Such behavior is disrespectful of one's self. If one cannot respect one's self, the unconscious family logic feels the same way.

Practice!

No! Have you ever noticed a two-year-old when they learn the word NO!? They love that word! "No" to a two-year-old means "My way, not your way." 'No' means the hatching into independence. "No" establishes the boundaries of self and not-self. "No" is a healthy way for the toddler to break away from the mother - infant FUSION. Healthy toddlers have a knack for saying 'no.' It is as if to say 'no' is a method of promoting self-discovery and growth. The co-dependent person can learn a lot from the toddler and begin the process of self-identity by simply saying, 'no.' For example, "No, I don't need your help on this, I can do this myself." Or, "No, this is something you need to learn how to do for yourself." In both of these examples we have seen now "no' works for the people-pleaser and the needy to establish independence OUT OF co-dependence.

Clarify

This does not mean we cannot do endearing things for each other. Far from it. The difference is this, when we do things for each other without patching a defect, we are grateful. Endearing jesters are like those nurturing notes or cards we give to each other. They are unexpected. However, when EXPECTED, the nurturing that is offered is received as a target of criticism, a form of entitlement. "You owe me, not enough…" rather then "That was so sweet, thank you!"

More thoughts on co-dependence

In a co-dependent relationship, there is really no satisfaction. Notice the prefix 'co' in co-dependence. This means that BOTH parties are psychological SLAVES to each other. It is like a freak of nature that both are joined in the mind by a delusion. One cannot go anywhere without the other psychologically. Where is the satisfaction in that? It is as if they are both psychological Siamese twins. To break apart would mean certain death to each delusional twin. However, with a bit of mind surgery (treatment), separation into independence may be achieved. Some surgery on twins are more dangerous than others. It just depends on how many psychological structures are co-habited and if the patient is willing to accept the risks in treatment for an independent and free life.

Should I?

Risk. Is independence worth the risk? If you think not, imagine being joined at the hip with a Siamese twin for life! If this is unacceptable, get a coach, (treater), learn to say 'no' and take a risk!

What is Projection, Exactly?

Written by Kathi Stringer

2/29/04

Projection is to blame another person for one's actions.
Primitive and Infantile Defense
In Adults: Chronic in most personality disorders

Projection – Action

You made me do it! Ever hear those words from an angry and frustrated child? In essence, the child is projecting the responsibility of his/her actions onto someone else. This child is anxious to rid themselves of the garbage. Projection is to 'blame' another. And, the words, 'you made me do it,' slip out ever so easily.

My little 5-year-old girl was listening to her grandparents in a tiff. Grandma said, "You made me [do this]!" Grandpa said, "No, you made me [make you do this]!" Finally, K, an intuitive child, shouted in response, "Stop projecting!" She caught them both by surprise. A small child had recognized projection in action.

Example: (Action)

Jim is holding an expensive camera. Jane is fumbling with the keys to the door. In the meantime, Jim drops and breaks the camera. Jim screams at Jane, "See what you made me do! I broke it because you didn't open the door!" Jim blamed Jane for dropping the camera. Jim could have prevented the camera from dropping if he had employed foresight and safety measures..i.e putting the camera band around his neck.

Projection – Emotional

You make me [feel] so mad! This is a bit more complicated because a degree of transference is involved. Easy speak - Transference = transferring memories from the past, placed onto a different person.

The derivatives of transference in this case transmutes into projection. Meaning, if an individual gets angry beyond the objective meaning of the statement, (reads more into it than intended) then a level of projection is at work. In other words, a person that reminds another individual of their hated father (transference at work - transference is ALWAYS a distortion), and OVERREACTS to a statement from that person based on that memory (triggered), then, that excessive anger would be projection.

Example: (Emotion)

Jane said, "Jim, just make a choice. We don't have all day." Jim screams back, "Why don't you just shut your big mouth?" and stormed off. On examination, Jim grew up with an over critical, and impatient mother. When Jane made her remark, Jim regressed into the child that hated his mother. Jim did not see Jane standing there at the moment. He saw his hated mother, in the transference. Now that Jim has a bigger body and is more confident to protect himself, he reacted in defense of the critical mother. It happened in a snap of the fingers. In this case, Jim was projecting out of his transference. Jim had distorted Jane into his hated mother. Remember, transference is always a distortion.

Caution:

While pointing out that action projection can be funny at times, *(Remark: You made me drop the hula-hoop when you spoke! – Response: ha ha projection!),* it is dangerous to point out the err of a person's behavior <u>during</u> an emotional projection, UNLESS YOU ARE A PROFESSIONAL. Since the person is caught up in the transference, empowered by the transference, and enraged by the transference, it would be wise to let the transference diminish before discussing the event. To address the distortion in the heat of the moment, can be perceived as minimizing the original trauma. This will lead to an unconscious perception of the invalidated child/victim (How dare you!? It did happen!). Wait until the person cools down and gets a grip back on reality and the transference is held in abeyance.

For Professionals:

The superlative therapeutic window to target projection, from the transference, would be in the height of the moment. However, a strong therapeutic alliance and rapport MUST BE established first. Trust is paramount. At this time, the client's internal closed core objects are 'hot' and can be redefined through a new experience. See more on 'projective identification.'

Projection Keyword Alerts

ACTION – You made me **do** it!
EMOTIONAL – You make me **feel** this way!

Question:

Is transference and projection the same?

Answer:

No. Some claim they are the same because psych can become convoluted (duh) to the point meanings are no longer clear to the novice. However, on exact examination, projection is 'caused' by the transference.

Transference is 'activated ***in*** the person, and ***projection*** is the release of that transference ***out of*** the person. *One treater said, "I hope you know, all this anger you are projecting on to me is not my anger, it is YOUR anger." The client coolly said, "Can you think of anything better to do with it?* (Gabbard)

Homework

Observe the number of times you can spot projection. Then, in cases of emotional projection, try to objectively determine the extent of the justified response vs. the transference reaction. Is if off just a little? Is it half-and-half? Is it way out there? This exercise can be a powerful indicator for self-awareness, an indicator to seek treatment for self or other.

References:

1. **Psych 101, Unlocking the Secret of Terms** - K. Stringer
   http://www.toddlertime.com/borderline/psych-101.htm

2. **An Object Relations Approach to Projective Identification and the Borderline** - K. Stringer
   http://www.toddlertime.com/borderline/projective.htm

3. **Star Trek and Projective Identification** - K. Stringer
   http://www.toddlertime.com/borderline/star-trek.htm

4. **Effective Inpatient Treatment And the Amelioration of the Therapeutic Alliance For Resistive Individuals with BPD** - K. Stringer
   http://www.toddlertime.com/borderline/alliance.htm

5. **Transference** - K. Stringer
   http://www.toddlertime.com/terms/transference.htm

6. **Defense Mechanisms** - K. Stringer
   http://www.toddlertime.com/terms/defense.htm

Transference

Written by Kathi Stringer

Transference is the patient's unrealistic projections onto the therapist. This consists of feelings and attitudes that were experienced previously from other persons in the patients life.

A given example is that the patient might get very angry with the therapist because prior feelings are resurrected, in that the doctor may be much like her mother, who stirred intense anger in her.

Transference is neither negative or positive. it is 'always a distortion.' A projection of emotions from the past to the current objects. (your doctor in this case)

Some transference issues are extremely inconsistent. For example, over-idealization (perceiving the therapist is all knowing) in transference can cause problems in a least two areas. (1) Since transference is the product of the patient's internal world, no person can actually fill that role, then along comes the disappointment, and rage, **or** (2) transference reaches into the patients world outside of the therapy office, others and relationships, and they not able to measure up to the projected transference of the therapist.

Transferences can also trigger sexual attraction by the patient. There are also psychotic transferences in which the patient doesn't observe the therapist as a representation of the object, but 'as the object.'

More on Transference

Psych 101 Unlocking the Secret of Terms

Effective Inpatient Treatment And the Amelioration of the Therapeutic Alliance for Resistive Individuals with BPD

Transitional Objects

Written by Kathi Stringer

Security

Usually in the first 5 to 18 months of age, the child may grow attached to a primary transitional object. Supplied and offered by mother, the object could be a blanket, diaper, teddy bear, bottle or other such similar article. The attachment is direct and not passive. The child's feelings for mother or primary caretaker spill over into the object which is used for self soothing and to reduce anxiety. Transitional objects acts as a substitutes, and bridge the representation of mother. For example - A child my curl up in mother's rocking chair when mother is not in the room for self comfort. This also an indication of a growing awareness that the child is separate from external objects and is an individual.

Blissful State

It is interesting that in tribal villages, the need for transitional objects are absent. This is because mother is always available to the toddlers. In western culture where the child sleeps in a different room, the transitional object helps ease the stress of separation. These objects provide security as they try to recapture the oneness of mother. At times a child my rock while holding the article projecting themselves into the blissful state of being held in mothers arms.

Holding Environment

Written by Kathi Stringer

This paper will attempt to discuss the analytic components of the holding environment and extrapolate theory to give meaning towards a syncretic result. First lets disassemble the codification of targeted principles to create a clear topographic model in this highly abstract concept. Winnicott, a British object relations theorist and pediatrician originated the "holding"(1960) and Bion (1967) the "containing" concepts. Stone (1981) goes on to say;

> "The "love" implicit in empathy, listening, and trying to understand, in nonseductive devotion to the task, the sense of full acceptance, respect, and sometimes the homely phenomenon of sheer dependable patience, may take their place as equal or nearly equal in importance to sheer interpretive skill. [p. 114]"

The holding and containing elements are particularly useful when treating regressive individuals with underdeveloped and disturbed object constancy common in the borderline. These clients employ infantile defense mechanisms, splitting, projective identification, denial, idealization and devaluation (Kernberg 1967). Integral of this process transferences will shift abruptly and so do their introspective of self (Mahler).

Boundaries

Writers (Scharff & Scharff, 1988) postulate the establishment of the holding environment must consist of boundaries. These include showing up for appointments on time, prompt payment and strict start and stopping times. Scharffs empathize these boundaries are needed to create a safe space in which the patient can feel protected, yet free to communicate, explore and experience. This modern psychology would seem self-defeating since to terminate a client due to trespassing over boundaries would allude to a presdo-holding environment since in truth the parallel would be to terminate a small child from the family relationship. Surely, exploration for alternate consequences for these regressed, self-sabotaging clients would prove advantageous for the therapeutic relationship. It would be imperative the treater not only be educated, but skilled and creative.

Containment

Lipthrott states that Bion (1967) developed concepts of the container and the contained both in therapy and in parenting. These terms of parenting, infants often become overwhelmed by affect because they lack the internal controls. The mothering caretaker pays attention, listens, takes in these communicated feelings whether they be cries, coos, laughter of facial expressions, transforms them, gives them meaning and returns them to the child resulting not only in necessary physical care for the child, but also an empathic soothing.

Holding Environment

Lipthrott also states that Winnicott speaks of a holding environment in which the infant is contained and experienced. The mother assists the child in the task of self-integration by reflecting back the child expression of him or herself. In his later writing, Winnicott describes mother functions as a mirror which provides the infant with "a precise reflection of his own experience and gestures, despite their fragmented and formless qualities."

Incomplete Therapy

Ninety percent of borderlines drop out of therapy (Kreisman 1991, p122). It is their primary nature to execute self-defeating behaviors and sabotage the therapeutic relationship. Like the toddler who runs from mother, expecting to be swooped up by her, she will instinctively test the safety capacity of her environment.

Self-defeating

The anaclitic quasi-symbiosis relationship with the therapist and treatment team will be under the scrutiny of the patient. In hopes to ameliorate her perception of the holding environment she will run like the toddler and dismiss those who are in a position to help her (such as case workers). Not game-playing but rather attempting to substantiate a consistent platform of trust and safety searching for the parental object. On the other hand, a patient may be so anaclitic depressed that the strength escapes her to proceed with therapy since she is incased with a shroud of helplessness and hopelessness. And finally, the patient when at odds with the world, who's behavior manifests negative transference will project her anger since she is unable to fulfill her notions, wishes and fantasies. Her fragile ego incapable of effectively using her previously maladaptive defense mechanisms will unconsciously elicit the same behavior she is projecting onto the therapist hoping to destroy the therapeutic stance and validate her perceptions of reality (the world is bad). In this instance the therapist should monitor her countertransference as a barometer to gage how the patient relates and responds to her internal structures and with others rather then in retaliation.

At any rate the therapy should continue as an open case for a period of supervision (telephone if necessary) to determine a definitive solution or hospitalization in a patient's failing mental health. A procedure short of this would damage the holding environment substantiating the patient's precarious fears of the vicissitudes of rejection and isolation.

Telephone strategies are a viable option to create and maintain an intrapsychic prophylaxis and a spatial element of the holding environment for the severely affected patient who is not able to operate. I formulate this conjecture to expand the therapist's modalities to reach beyond the static office climate into the patient's world of the here-and-now. This therapeutic tool may mitigate and stifle the growing anxiety of rejection and abandonment, giving rise to object constancy, bringing escalating emotions into manageable proportions. Such tactics will inhibit the neurotic rapture of desperation in the borderline.

More on the Holding Environment

Holding Environment for the Borderline

An Object Relations Approach to Understanding Unusual Behaviors and Disturbances

Psych 101 - Unlocking the Secret of Terms

Fundamentals of Splitting

Written by Kathi Stringer

Individuals who have not achieved object constancy /object permanence still relate to reality using the defensive of splitting. They are unable the identify the feelings of others and view them objectively.
An infant fears that once mother is out-of-sight, she is destroyed, not having the capacity to visualize a permanent image of her. This can be demonstrated by the developmental tool of a game called, peak-a-boo. When the hands of mother are pulled away, viewing her face, the infant is delighted and saddened when not in view.
Adults who are splitting relate much in the same way that the infant sees reality as all-good or all-bad with polarized view points. The mental representations of good and bad are not integrated and prevents them from seeing the one they destroy is the same one who soothes and comforts. They do not have a tolerance of loving and hating toward the same person, unable to see them as some good and some bad. They cannot tolerate ambivalence hence the term, splitting.

The individual who causes the frustration is seen as all bad, and if pleasurable, then all good. In the same way, these traits are often seen with those who are depressed one minute and elated the next. This behavior can be seen in toddlers who throw temper tantrums. The toddler is frustrated with both poles of thought, dependence / independence and hate / love.

For this reason the parent / therapist would do well to provide a "holding environment" and contain the unintegrated feelings, metabolize them and give meaning. Once they have the cognitive equipment and skills, able to achieve object constancy, then the internal struggle is relieved. Ultimately, client / toddler needs to experience the good-enough-partner / good-enough-mother while holding feelings of "bad" primarily toward that object.

Since the therapist / mother is not always available, the client / toddler needs to find other ways to internally soothe and comfort, then entering into the transitional process. The effect must be experienced in doses in which the client / toddler can handle them.

More Written on Splitting

Psych 101 - Unlocking the Secret of Terms

Effective Inpatient Treatment And the Amelioration of the Therapeutic Alliance for Resistive Individuals with BPD
Treatment Strategies with Borderline Personality Clients

Thoughts on Projective Identification

Written by Kathi Stringer

I think the most deadly of all projections is projective identification (PI). Usually due to the subject being invalidated to some degree, the subject will lash out at the invalidating/misunderstanding treater (or S/O, nurse, staff, friend..etc). This lashing out consists of, for example, the splitting-off of the bad-object, say anger in this case, and projecting that anger into the target/treater. Of course since every treater reacts different depending on their countertransference hook, the subject may have to keep projecting modified objects until the treater accepts the projection. Then wham! We have projective counter-identification (PCI), in which the treater has accepted the projected object and is now identifying with that object. The pay-off for the subject is some element of control.i.e.."now I can make you feel as bad as you made me feel." All the while the treater now feels as though some alien took over their essence and is miserable. Pay back...so it seems. This unconscious goal for the subject was to race for the high ground and identify with the abuser and NOT the victim. As we all know, in the either/or domain of splitting, there is only an abuser or a victim, and no middle ground. The beat up subject that is flooded with emotions and not able to tolerate/hold the frustration will project the uncomfortable material via projective identification as a HOT POTATO. This all happens unconsciously, like, SNAP. The treater is now in the victim role, and the subject is at the controls, it feels like some sort of revenge in the transference.

Yet, what comes next separates the difference between a professional handing PI and an amateur treater, or some dip on the psych unit.

The Fundamentals of the Transitional Phenomena

Written by Kathi Stringer

Winnicott has termed an area between fantasy and reality as the *potential space* in which the two rendezvous without consequences. How is this safe area possible? Let's first examine dynamics of the transitional object.

The infant or toddler in his first true creative act will imbue an object with symbolic meaning as a defensive measure to carry-over the presence of mother or primary caretaker. This object is *created* by the baby and the acceptance of a symbol and is usually in the concrete form of a blanket, diaper or such soft article and usually represents mother's maternal presence and softness. This aids the baby in the transition of relating to omniavailable mother as differentiated from self and others. Hence the term, Transitional Object.

Since the baby is still using splitting as a primary defensive mechanism, he is unable to integrate the idea that mother's love still exists when unavailable. Subsequently, the transitional object performs as bridge as it will serve to comfort the baby until he can comprehend his reality in more abstract terms. In this way, the baby manipulates his *possession*, a part of himself and mother.

Later, concrete object transitions will move into the abstract transitional phenomena. This is an interim region between fantasy / reality and omnipresence / objectively. This *potential space* is what Winnicott viewed as play, an infinite intermediate area where external and internal reality are amalgamated. Correspondingly, this is a territory in which the subject can take on the identity of a fictional character interlaced with his own identity without fear or retaliatory consequences. It is though this *play* that one can explore and perceive self and his relation to others.

It has been speculated and argued quiet successfully that the *potential space* in the therapist office is play / illusion, (Illusion is a derived from the root, . in- + ludere, to play). This is seen and understood as the exchange / dialectic, the exploration between therapist and client in the safety of the office. On a higher, more sophisticated level, cultural and societal components enter into the transitional process in determining identity of self.

What is Ego-Syntonic?

Question:

I'm seeking to find information on the meaning of the terms 'ego-syntonic' and 'ego-dystoni'. I wonder if you can help please.

Answer:

In short,

- syntonic= behaviors "insync" with the ego (no guilt)
- dystonic= behavior "dis-n-sycn' with the ego (guilt)

The ego's job is to determine the best course of action based on information from the ID, reality, and the Super Ego (SE). When the ego is comfortable with it's conclusions and behaviors, (in denial in these sort of cases), one is said to be ego-syntonic. For example, an individual with borderline personality disorder (BPD) that is in denial, could be an ego-syntonic BPD. However, if the person with BPD were bothered by some of their behaviors, they would be an ego-dystonic BPD.

Understanding
Borderline Personality Disorder (BPD)

i. Personal Insight
ii. Letters/Questions and Understanding BPD
iii. Clinical Therapeutic Models for Individuals with BPD

Section i

"Personal Insight "

Why I Research

Written by Kathi Stringer
December 12, 2003

Hey gang, just a bit about your website Host. I get letters wondering about 'me.' I've evaded them for years, but what the heck. So tonight I decided to tap out the ASCII, to write what I feel, and when I feel it.

It's the holidays. I've been hospitalized 3 times in the last 30 days and over 30 times since 1996. Yes, I understand about triggers. Yet, I take responsibility by acknowledging 'it's me' not just the triggers. I've been dx'd as borderline personality disorder severe more times than I can count fingers. It is a perplexing diagnosis since on personality instrument scales it shows that I do not have the traits to be labeled with any AXIS II disorder. Of course, with my knowledge in mental health and psychology, it isn't hard to figure out which sort of questions applies to which personality disorder. Question: "Do you have inappropriate anger?" Flash for the scorekeeper…my mind registers, borderline personality disorder question! Duh! I guess you could say that I beat the tests. It's hard to answer those type of instruments honestly when my intellect is a defense guarding my raw emotions. It's bad enough I have emotional problems that I will not show stupidly.

I had seen different practitioners that dispute whether I have BPD or PTSD/ Bipolar. Frankly, when I get caught up into the 'emotions' I really don't see choice on how I relate to the world, or nor do I care what the dx is. My emotions go to autopilot. And, I do regress and 'fast.' I function emotionally as a toddler. I don't 'act out' but rather 'act in.' This is the strange part. I've been self-employed since I was 23-years-old, and I built my company as key supplier for Hughes Aircraft when I reached age 26. I have only a 10th grade education. Some psychologists say my intellect is high, and I quote, "high enough to flip into craziness or do great things." I think more toward craziness myself. With intellect, things come easy. With emotions, I'm lost and completely clueless when I get caught up 'into it.' There are times when I've been challenged to change my behavior when 'in it.' And you know what? I usually become defensive. I can out-solve my accuser on an intellectual platform in areas they look like idiots, so…how dare they point out my emotional weakness when I'm not rude to call them an idiot? It seems sort of one-sided at times.

I'm emotionally arrested due to the same-ole-stuff. Child abuse. Bad stuff. I had to fake at being an adult to take care of my brothers and sister. My emotional progress got fixated since I suddenly had to pretend 'not to be me' anymore. I had to 'act' big and take care of things, and all while dealing with blood stained walls. So, does this etiology appear as PTSD or the precursor makings of borderline personality disorder? Well, when 'locked in,' it really doesn't matter. It is another world all together.

So, why do I write all the scientific material about mental health? During one of my first inpatient stays I was pretty wasted by staff. So much so, that I went to the city college and bought every psych book they had. My mind began getting interested in solving what the hell was going on with me, and why and the hell I was treated so badly (revenge). Within months my interested turned to the professional publishers –ARONSON and the APA. I invested thousands of dollars in publications, journals and scholarly books. In BPD books alone, my collection is upwards from 40 of them. Not the pop psych in the 'self-improvement' section at the bookstore, but hard-core theory – Searles, Adler, Paris, Gabbard, Kernberg, Gunderson, Volkan, Chatham, Linehan, Silk, Goldstein, Sherwood, Cohen, Chessick, Masterson, Robson, Meissner, Hartocollis…just in BPD, not including the hundreds of other books in object relations and related supporting psych. I was out to get armed with knowledge to prevent future abuses from mental health. And you know what I learned? How to say the 'golden rule' in extreme and convoluted psych format. Then, and only then would I be taken seriously. For example, if I were to say, "ouch, that hurt" I would get a list of coping skills with blame at my feet. Now, with this education, I can say something like, "ouch, try a little countertransference management please?" and that sinks in. And, it really bugged me that I needed to go to such extremes just to be 'safe' so that I could tell the difference what was 'proto-call' and what was just plain being mean in staff attitudes.

Now I know the difference, and I no longer have to doubt myself. Since, I've turned this knowledge to my website as an outreach to other mental health providers. The revenge subsided and was replace with an honest and sincere effort to make a connection with providers. To share what I've learned from my experience combined with my studies. I suppose in making the 'connection' I lose some of my readers without a psych background. I choose those with a psych background because that is where my raw 'wounds' are. I needed to address much of the stereotyping about BPD 'mental patient's' and those that are fixated from early emotional trauma.

Lets take a look at borderline personality disorder vs PTSD for a second. When I was inpatient and a mental health worker said to me, "STEP AWAY FROM THE RED LINE!" I turned and saw the MHW was speaking to me. Instantly, the back of my neck 'warmed' and I felt like I was caught back up in the battle zone of childhood memories. His demandingness came across as the abusive father that beat and screamed. In a split second all my logic, and presence-of mind-vanished. I was looking at an abuser. I was looking at a HATED abuser. And, I screamed back, "OR WHAT??" I was triggered. I went into autopilot. The child woke up and refused to be abused any longer. Then the MHW said, "OR YOU WILL END UP IN SECLUSION AND RESTRAINTS!" Ouch. The abusive environment has challenged me. The child was aroused. The intellect became useless. The emotions were much to important to be denied, not now, not after all the denial that came from childhood, no…not now. I ended up in seclusion and restraints.

Now, does it really matter that it was borderline personality disorder or PTSD? I suppose it can be argued. The point is, at that moment, I was lashing back at an abuser in the transference. And, how powerful that connection can be. Massive.

Today I'm still struggling with those inpatient nightmares that woke up the abused child. And, I thought, what the hell, I'll write you, and maybe, just maybe we might have something in common. I really do understand. I too am vulnerable, but I try to put up a stiff upper lip. We, you and me, we are survivors, else we wouldn't be here. Yes, I have my fun with the BPD page…. but I suppose there could be a lot of anger in reverse. It is my way of sharing the 'maddness' the 'hopelessness' and the anger. Anger inward.

You know, just an added thought. I could never figure out why God let Jesus die…all that blood. Now I understand, 'someone' had to pay, even if an innocent. With BPD's and PTSD that act-in, someone has to pay, and it is us. Now, finally, I get the concept.

My BPD Symptoms

Written by Kathi Stringer

Brief symptoms and diagnostic criteria for Borderline Personality Disorder, for Kathi Stringer

Must meet 5 of 9 for BPD

1. Avoid Abandonment (**Yes**)

2. Unstable Relationships (**No**)

3. Identity Disturbance (**Yes**)

4. Impulsively - self damaging (**Yes**) Spending & Starvation

5. Suicidal Ideation or self-mutilating behavior (**Yes**) Feel like an alien on the wrong planet and act-in from deep depression of seeing the real world.

6. Mood Swings (**Yes**) maybe bi-polar trait

7. Chronic feelings of emptiness (**Yes**) Cannot feel enough goodness from the world since the internal good object is not there from abusive childhood and verified from treatment in the hospital.

8. Inappropriate anger (**No**)

9. Severe dissociative symptoms (**Yes**)

So, I guess that makes 7 of 9. I only wish I were 7-of-9 from Voyager!

JUDGEMENT DAY

Mixed State

People with Bipolar Disorder can experience a mixed state that is probably the most painful and potentially lethal bipolar condition as well as the most difficult to treat.

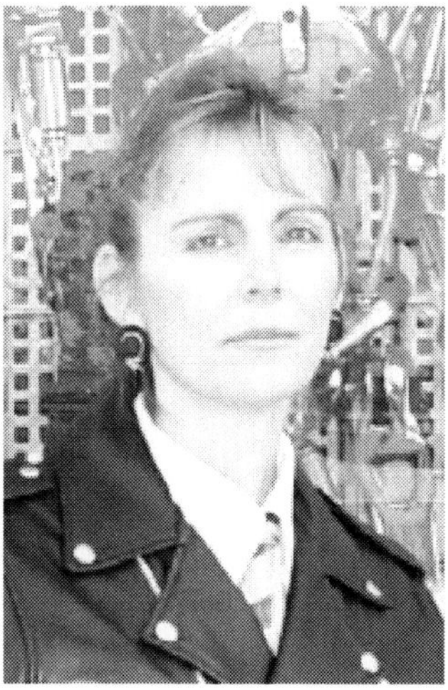

Kathi Stringer - Judgment Day
March 15, 2001

Judgment Day

The picture on the left, and one right below, were taken on March 15, 2001 - Judgment Day. It was a day that I set aside for judging whether to stay on this planet because I was becoming more and more despondent over depressive ruminations from abuse by Riverside County Mental Health & Richard Dorsey AKA; RGH.

Variations -
The Harvard Mental Health Letter -
Mixed State - April 2001

Mixed State

Many people also suffer residual symptoms between episodes of depressions and mania, moods that cycle rapidly in bursts, or - in many ways, worst of all - a mixed state in which they are energetic, hyperactive, and sleepless, and at the same time angry, irritable, and despondent. Their racing thoughts are filled with depressive ruminations, and their decreased need for sleep (typical of mania) becomes insomnia (typical of depression). This mixed state is probably the most painful and potentially lethal bipolar condition as well as the most difficult to treat. It is the mood in which a person with bipolar disorder is most likely to commit suicide.

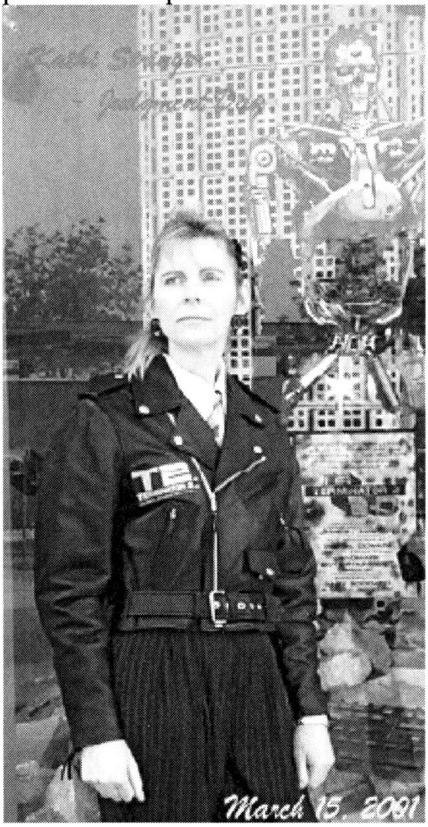

Judgment Day

Written on March 17, 2001

Judgment Day - A day I set aside to determine if the pain of life was worth its rewards. It's no wonder that I went for a personal visit to the site of the Terminator. I was filled with anger, and depression, and to terminate the situation seemed the likely choice.

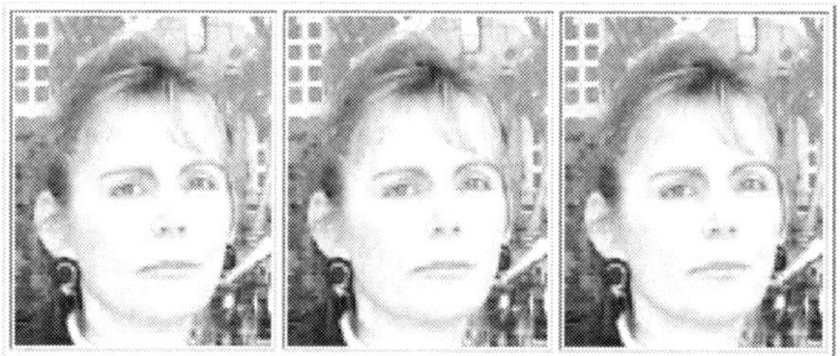

Mixed - Most painful and potentially lethal

1996

I was hospitalized by RGH (Riverside General Hospital) and during this admit, I was laughed at and made the butt-end of cruel jokes. This admit and those that followed awakened symptoms of Post Traumatic Stress Disorder (PTSD), and Bipolar Disorder. Once these symptoms were awakened, a reverberation of these two disorders would feed off each other, then geometrically crystallize into a new model, shifting it's shape to elude doctors. The dynamics were hidden behind a maze of flashbacks fueled with anger and frustration that gave way to more severe methods of self-attack.

1998

It has been 2 years now and the abuse by RGH still continued. It was an endless cycle similar to the Bipolar disorder itself with its extreme poles of emotion and thought; - provoked by mistreatment. It was like the electronic sine wave with anger peaks and depression valleys. Once I would be released from RGH, I would reflect on the abusive treatment and sink into a depression which lead to behaviors for rehospitalization. Once rehospitalized, I could not work on my own issues because I was caught up into senseless power struggles, and hatred toward a system that testified to a Judge that my periods of regression was repulsive to staff.

1998

I filed lawsuit against the Medical Director and RGH. The hospitalizations still continued. The Riverside County Board of Supervisors hired attorneys to block the suit and defend the ubiquitous abuse.

1999-2000

In conjunction with the shape-shifting constellation of PTSD and Bipolar Disorder, I now had to face the anxiety from depositions and discovery. Think of this anxiety as the accelerator to boost levels of the present agitated symptoms. The 3 of them in the mixing pot, PTSD, Bipolar and fueled by anxiety produced a Bipolar Mixed State that is probably the most painful and potentially lethal bipolar condition as well as the most difficult to treat.

A Superior Court Judge remarked in court that in his view the law gave immunity to RGH and my patient's rights' meant nothing. The Judge said, yes, my rights were violated,.... but immunity,.... there are immunities. This shocking revelation sent me into a downward spiral of anger. How dare they? I was abused as a child and now even as an adult - after handling the situation appropriately through the court channels, the abuse received immunity. How dare they?!

2001

January 2, 2001 - The last months my life thus far had been an array of frustrated and angry depressed thoughts. A jury would not hear my testimony. My present symptoms are still not diagnosed. [Worst of all - a mixed state in which they are energetic, hyperactive, and sleepless, and at the same time angry, irritable, and despondent. My racing thoughts were filled with depressive ruminations.] I remembered the austere imprint of being in a brighter mood to suddenly without warning turn to tears and feeling as though I would sink into the earth. I remembered falling down to my knees in a crushing motion, now in a frustrated upright fetal position and then jerk my head straight up and scream, "God, what's wrong with me??!!! I can't do this anymore, I HATE THIS!" I have been complaining now for some months to most of my friends how "painful" my life is in regards to sleep deprivation, mind numbing and tingling.

Then - the eluding mixed state cornered me and I was seemly without an advocate. At this point I didn't know anything about a Bipolar Mixed State and believed my thoughts that centered around abuse (PTSD) would prevent me from ever living a normal life again, that is the ruminations of the abuse from RGH. How I hated those flashbacks, those thoughts. In the late hours of the night I would try and lie down hoping for sleep, and what a joke that was. My brain was tingling, yes, tingling, numbed and zombied out, and yet I STILL could not sleep! I was like the living UNDEAD! I might as well be dead!

It was getting late into the evening. I had it. I had made a decision to cut. Cutting myself meant getting this blood out of me that I no longer considered my own. RGH turned me into something else besides myself. This blood-letting would be a symbolic cleansing and also serve to make the UNDEAD, DEAD. I began cutting...

> Police Report - "I noticed that Ms. Stringer had a lot of dried blood on the right side of her neck and throat.....I told Ms. Stringer to put down the razor blade. She continued to cut at her wrist...Just shoot me, why don't you....just go ahead and shoot me."

The police were trying to save me and I was angry. I did not see this as help but to only prolong the situation. I was out of it.

FEB 2001

In the weeks that followed, I was still not diagnosed as this mixed-state. If you can believe this, I went to court from the hospital and fought hard for the 'right-to-die'. With the judge's final words, he echoed that his decision could be seen as cruel but he could not allow me to end my life, thereby committing me for a hospitalization term of up to 180 days. I was there less then 2 weeks because of my personal written commitments, and that got me off the hook. I was freed again.

Judgment Day Set

Days later I offset my date to March 15, 2001 - Judgment Day, to decide if I wanted to stay on this same piece of dirt as all those who got immunity for abusing me. I was going to weigh it all out. This may sound silly to you, but to me it was serious. Most of the people at RGH, all 3 shifts had their 'fun way', and evil comments. And to be a part of that cultural base, to experience what society offered toward recovery, meant to endorse the abuse I went through as a child. I thought humans were better then that, trained better, and cared more, yet it was repeated all over again, the childhood abuse - the there-and-then into the here-and-now.

Toward Judgment Day I received altruistic endeavors from nurses, doctors, friends and family. Pat (a friend) came to visit me every single day while I was in the hospital with Trish in tow most of the time. I remembered Brad an RN from a wonderful hospital that began the collection with, "Kathi, you are a beautiful Child of God." I took this single phrase along with Dr. Witkowski's helpful remarks that - "It is okay to be who I am and so what if I am different?" Yet, even though I had all this, it wasn't enough as I still had too many days & nights as the UNDEAD - the dreaded mixed bipolar state. My thoughts had me caught up in a chemical imbalance that reverberated between my brain tingling and a sea of brooding emotions. At this time I was lost. I had no way to understand any of this. Why am I the living UNDEAD?

FEB 2001 - Light

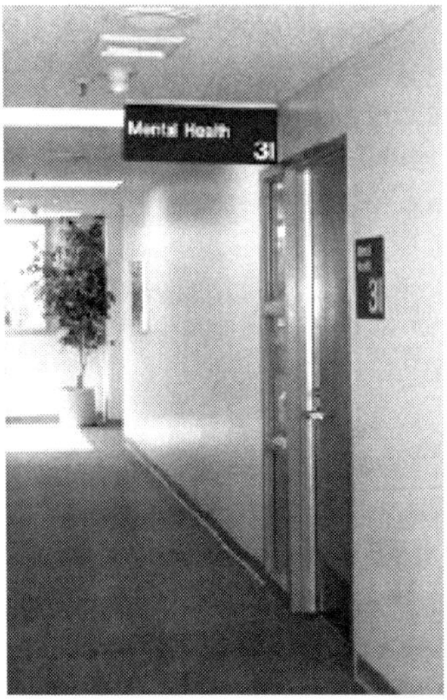

Dr. Witkowski (Kaiser) begins to recognize bipolar symptoms and a possible mixed state. She gave me information to digest but I only skimmed through it, at this point I was burned out on learning any new in-depth mental health junk. So, I did what any good sister would do, I faxed it to my baby brother and asked him to read through all of it and explain it to me. And he did exactly that! Family support! It takes a lot for a family remember to sit down, take the time and read this stuff, but he did, and that meant a lot to me. My brother spoke with me after researching this stuff and we hashed it out as team players. That was an important concept - team players.

My friends supported me in the same way. Patty, web owner of Mental Health Sanctuary, who also has this bipolar disorder, swung into action and painfully wrote and rewrote a letter to me, basically telling me "to get the hell out of my own way." Patty's letter affected me so much that I dreamt about it that night. That letter is here.

So far what was explained to me was about the bipolar state. I was 'trying' to accept that, but I was having trouble. Then it happened, the ballpark flood-lights came on when a Harvard Mental Health Letter that I subscribed to came across my desk. That month's volume and issues dealt with Bipolar Disorder - Part 1. It was there that I read the paragraph above describing the bipolar mixed state. Bingo, that was it, that was me!

Knowledge is power. I now have hope that perhaps my brain may one day work correctly together with it's neurotransmitters and dissolve this horrible bipolar mixed state.

So whatever happened to Judgment Day? I don't know. My friends didn't give me a chance to reflect and make that judgment. They surrounded me that day and we stayed busy. I feel like I got jip out of something and didn't get the chance to follow through. It has only been 2 days now, so lets see how it goes from here......

Thank you for hanging with me during this long painful journey that has yet to be concluded. If you have any comments or similar stories, it would be great if you allowed me to post them here. Be sure to read the summary below.

SUMMERY - Bipolar Mixed-State

1. The correct diagnosis is very important toward recovery. My brother said I should "kiss my doctor" for figuring this one out ;-)

2. The establishment of a positive therapeutic team alliance with your doctor, nurse and therapist will promote wellness.

3. Getting more then an "ahhhh, poor baby" and real family support with research and reading is very helpful.

4. True friends are cool. They didn't run but rather got into the meat of the matter. They put up with my abusing irritations and watched me abuse myself, and they still stuck. Friends look toward solutions, not pity. Friends, period.

Put this all together and I have a good chance toward recovery.

The War Machine and Mental Health

Written by Kathi Stringer

***Cavort*:** The mental health system implied represents inpatient treatment at Riverside General Hospital (RGH).

The War Machine

The US got together it's very best to formulate, build and train an effective war machine to eradicate, annihilate and erase opposing forces. This machine was the construct from endorsements of the Senate, Congress and Assemblyman. This embodiment represents our elected officials and so elected by the good faith of the majority of citizens of America to carry forth the will and intent of American people. Therefore, the actions and effectiveness of the war machine may be viewed as a representation of the institutions and ideologies that created and endorsed it.

Basically, that said, the direction and attitudes of the war machine reflect directly on those that created it. The will, morals and ethical virtues of this Nation are the foundation from which this war machine is firmly rooted.

Succinctly, the war machine is a probable reflection of the beliefs and attitudes of the majority of the American people. The machine was well thought out, well structured, well designed, well trained and highly effective. The war machine takes care of business and does what it was designed for -- to protect the security of the United States.

The Mental Health System

After pondering the strength and effectiveness of the war machine and linking that effectiveness with the American people, why then should the mental health delivery system be viewed any differently? After all, those that run the system were trained by our institutions, and we as a nation decided what knowledge, tone and attitude should passed onto its students. One has to assume we are using our best trainers and thinkers of our time to set into motion a care system that is healing and compassionate for the people it represents. Ourselves.

My Experience

When hospitalized, I was called 'crazy', 'coo coo' and repulsive by a multicultural and multidisciplinary treatment team that encompassed three shifts of people. In my mind this team represented those that trained, supported and empowered them. Mainly, my society. Society has put its essence into the framework of the vocational system to reflect the concerns of its citizens.

So, when I am asked, "How does what happened to me have anything to do with the rest of society outside the mental health system?" I answered, "Because the mental health system was trained to heal. They were trained to put its best foot forward, and if this is its best, to reflect on me so poorly, demeaning and contemptuous, then I am an alien and truly am on the wrong planet. The mental health system as done what it has been designed to do, and I have felt it. They have said I was repulsive and defective."

The Aftermath

Now, I feel angry and behind that anger is hurt, sadness and disappointment. I feel like I'm not worth the trouble to be nurtured. I feel like my feelings are bizarre and without merit. The mental health system taught me this and our governing agencies and the Constitution supported their position.

I feel rebellious. I feel they are wrong -- or -- if they are right, then I have no worth, because that which I hold dear, my child alter is repulsive and all I ever wanted was to be loved, loved for my true-self and not the false masque that I hide behind to protect myself from hurtful faces.

The American people have their war machine to protect them.

They are protected.

I have the mental health system to protect me. If this is truly protection, then I will forever wonder about the feelings of safety, validation and nurturing. Because I have been stripped and raped of my true-self. It has been cast aside and found repulsive.

I feel lost, confused and hopeless.

Who am I?

They are repulsed by what is behind the masque.

They say it is a delusion.

Then my true-self is a delusion.

Then I truly am an alien on the wrong planet. I am not me, only who I pretend to be. They want their Pretender, not me.

Borderline Personality Disorder:

The Basic Five

Written by Kathi Stringer

If you have been diagnosed with Borderline Personality Disorder or care about someone with Borderline Personality Disorder, then this site is for you. Begin with reading **Borderline Personality Disorder: Day One**, written by a person that was diagnosed with Borderline Personality Disorder.

You have just been diagnosed with Borderline Personality Disorder (BPD) and you're perhaps wondering exactly what is Borderline Personality Disorderand what to expect from your treater. This is a good place to start. As you begin your journey, there are 5 basic things you need to know in order begin recovery. Once we are finished, I will help you get more of what you need to know.

ONE

Focus on knowledge, commitment and attitude. This is important. Learn everything you can about Borderline Personality Disorder. Kathi's Mental Health Review can help you do that. Another good source for some basic information is written in a book called, "I Hate You, Don't Leave Me." It's cheap. Get it.

It is hard to recover from Borderline Personality Disorder but not impossible. It takes a firm commitment on your part. Statistics are against you because most individuals with Borderline Personality Disorder drop out of treatment and continue to victimize them selves. This is why it is important to stay focused and committed. Your treater, best friend, family and support system are great for knowledge and guidance, but in reality you must make this journey alone. It would be like working out; only the person lifting the weight is going to get the most benefit.

Keep a good attitude. In the beginning and during the recovery process you may regress with setbacks. This is to be expected. When this happens don't be too hard on yourself. The mistake is not from falling down, but from not getting back up again.

TWO

Find a good therapist. This is most important. Some therapists won't work with Borderline Personality Disorder because it drains them, so ask about this right up front. Remember, the therapist is not there to be your buddy and best friend, but to challenge you. Evidence shows that a therapist that specializes in Borderline Personality Disorder will help you get better, faster. If you have your therapist wrapped around your finger, then it's time to move on. You are just wasting your money and your time.

Ask a lot of questions about your care. It's okay to disagree with a treatment strategy. It is okay to be a part of the decision making process so when the plan is set into motion you will feel comfortable and compliant. After all, it's your mental health at stake, not theirs.

THREE

Don't be afraid of change. It is okay to have Borderline Personality Disorder. What is not okay is too accept it without motivation for change. People in general hate change. Jack that up 1000% for individuals with Borderline Personality Disorder. If you lose your focus, and remember nothing else, remember this; you need to change for the healing process to begin.

FOUR

You are not your illness. Rather you are a unique individual with Borderline Personality Disorder. So don't beat yourself up for this. Treaters tend to generalize when speaking about Borderline Personality Disorder behaviors. To meet the Borderline Personality Disorder criteria as outlined in the DSM IV-R, your treater's reference book, you must at least meet 5 of the 9 symptoms. You may meet only 5 or all 9 in the severest form. This translates into 156 different variations for Borderline Personality Disorder and each may present much differently to a treater. Keep this in mind when you search for knowledge since some information may not apply to your particular symptoms.

FIVE

Get a good support system, a network. The worst thing you can do is put the full load on a single person. Spread it out because they won't be able to handle it and will burnout. That will make you feel worse. Set up a plan for when certain feelings begin to overwhelm you because sometimes a person with Borderline Personality Disorder can't do it alone.
There is also support on the Internet. You will meet folks that can listen and validate what you are going trough. It can also provide a forum of you to journal. However, you should also know the pitfalls from this type of support. Be careful from falling into the trap of becoming the Borderline Personality Disorder identity. Some individuals don't want to get better and hang onto Borderline Personality Disorder because without it they will feel emptier.

These are the Basic 5. Keep them handy. Be good to yourself and give yourself a hug from time to time. If you find that you are knee-deep in self-pity for a few days, that's fine but remember to snap out of it.

Borderline Personality Disorder Pathology and Treatment

Written by Kathi Stringer

Revision A. 8/25/03

As a cavort, I would like to suggest that borderline pathology is *not* the fault of the client because she has not fully reached certain developmental levels. Instead, she has relied on a maze of mental structures and primitive defense mechanisms that contributed to her cognitive dissonance. Yet, I firmly believe that a treater working with a multidisciplinary team conducting a carefully selected treatment plan that could, validate, modify, limit, empathize and provide a *holding environment*, might reverse what others criticize as the chronic personality disorder. By employing methods of genuine concern and strong countertransference management, the unattainable may be attained.

The indented purpose of this work is to discuss Borderline Personality Disorder (BPD) and its vicissitudes within its respective spectrum. Borderline has long been a controversial label. It was once thought to be denoted some where between psychosis and neurosis (Stern, 1938; Kernberg, 1975). Because of the inconsistency of BPD, professionals have had a hard time setting the criteria for this personality disorder. At one time, BPD was informally used, a catch-all, garbage-can diagnosis for individuals who did not fit into more characteristic diagnostic slots. It wasn't until 1980 that BPD was included into the DSM III. Five of the eight must be present to meet the criteria for BPD, although, the risk of suicide increases with each inclusion. Note* DSM IV [2] added an extra criteria, #9.

1. Frantic efforts to avoid real or imagined abandonment.

2. Unstable and intense interpersonal relationships. One moment they may idealize their partner, the next, completely devaluate them. (example of splitting)

3. Identity is always in question. Unstable self-image and sense of self. Borderlines have even been know to change their gender in search of self.

4. Impulsiveness. At least in two areas and are self damaging. Such areas include; gambling, sex, reckless driving, spending sprees, binge eating, drugs & etc.

5. Suicidal ideation. Self-mutilating, gestures, threats and behavior. Starvation. (in some cases, this is not to die, but to feel something, anything, to feel alive.)

6. Severe mood shifts. Depressed and lost one moment and euphoric the next.

7. Chronic feelings of emptiness and boredom. Life is generally uninteresting and holds no meaning.

8. Inappropriate display of anger, or difficulty controlling anger, temper tantrums.

9. Stress-related paranoid ideation. Severe dissociate symptoms.

Inclusive, there is empirical evidence pointing to a high comorbidity of transient major depression and axis two Borderline Personality Disorder. Also, 1.8% to 4% of the general population have Borderline Personality Disorder and the female to male ratio is 3:1. The percentage rises with inpatient at 23% and outpatient at 11%.

The preferred treatment modality used by professionals include three components; individual psychotherapy, group therapy and medication. Medication plays an significant role in recovery since 90% of the time medication is used during treatment. It is important that the psychiatrist and psychotherapist keep the lines of communication open to stifle the common countertransference problems in the area.

Two major forms of psychotherapies are used with treatment of the borderline. One is Dialectal Behavior Therapy or DBT (Linehan, 1993) [3] and Psychodynamic Psychotherapy (Kernberg, 1989). First, lets enumerate the principles of psychodynamic therapy and then elaborate further.

Stability of the framework of treatment.

- Borderline clients do very well with structure.
- Increased activity of the therapist.
- Tolerance of the patient's hostility without retaliating or withdrawing.
- Making self-destructive behaviors ungratifying.
- Focusing on connection between actions and feelings.
- Setting limits - Blocking acting-out behaviors that threaten the safety of the patient, the therapist or the therapy.
- Focus clarifications and interpretations on the here-and-now.
- Careful monitoring of counter-transference feelings.

Minimize Silence

The treater would do well to facilitate the session to minimize silence since it does not go over well with the client. For example (Gabbard) [1], the treater might say, "You are quiet, would you share with me what you are thinking?" or, "I have a feeling that something is troubling you, and you seem to be sorting it out." or "I noticed with my last remark, you became quiet." This is important to help decrease the risk of the client interpreting the silence as uncaring, callus and cold.

Primary Effect, Anger

The clear and constant hallmark of the borderline is the ubiquitous anger and rage, the primary effect. It would be advantages for the treater to tolerate the project anger, then identify and contain it, rather then retaliating or withdrawing which would impede the therapeutic environment. Working with the borderline triggers countless countertransference problems. The emergence of countertransference stems from the debilitating behavior of the borderline who is unable to function, evoking intense feelings of anger from the therapist.

Link Consequence to Event

The treater should identify the sympathetic elements of self-destructive action that transmutes to consequences. Some of these destructive behaviors are bingeing, self-mutation, self-destructive behavior in interpersonal relationships, suicide gestures to self-bullying. For example, a client may not realize self-mutation is not recognized in society as normal, and has a direct consequence. In the borderline, it is not uncommon for them to have split-off the interpsychic process of "action equals consequence."

Impulsiveness

The unequivocal identification of the borderline is their impulsiveness. They have a tendency to react, rather then to respond. They compartmentalize their unintegrated thoughts, preventing them from making the connection of rational choices. They are completely unaware that events-feelings-behavior are interrelated. For example, Jim told his therapist that he went out and got drunk last night for no apparent reason. He didn't know why. Exploring this further, earlier that day, Jim had won a class award for which he did not feel worthy. His low self esteem turned to guilt which led to his impulse to drink. Linking these intrinsic factors (events-feelings-behavior) will provide a cathexis to ameliorate cognitive correction, the ability to respond.

Address the Here-and-Now

Given the complex ideology, fifty to seventy percent of borderlines experienced childhood abuse, neglect and trauma. All to often the borderline tends to drudge up the past, exposing buried relics in preference of dealing with the problems of the here-and-now. I am not suggesting their childhood should not be reexamined for relevance to current behaviors, by all means it should be, but rather held in abeyance while dangerous, current inappropriate behaviors are dealt with. For example, Ricky is constantly getting into fights at school and destroying school property. The immediate situation calls for improved coping skills and a plan to advert his reactions to negative stimuli. Now lets turn to:

General principles of Dialectical Behavior Therapy (Linehan) [3]

Once weekly group and once weekly individual therapy

Primary impairment is reviewed as a constitutional dysregulation of control of emotion and effect

A number of behavioral outcomes are identified that result from this underlying difficulty.

Group therapy teaches patients behavioral coping skills.

Individual therapy focuses on 6 goals

Suicidal behaviors

Therapy - Interfering behaviors

Behaviors that interfere with the quality of life.

Behavioral skill acquisition

Posttraumatic stress behaviors

Self-respect behaviors

Suicidal Ideation

According to Linehan [3], parasuicide or suicide crisis behaviors should be taken seriously and I must agree. According to research, seven to ten percent of borderlines kill themselves. When in session a treater might determine when the thought entered the client's mind. For example, the treater could ask what set off the feelings of suicide. At times, a borderline will want to make an impact and erroneously think that her death would severely disrupt the therapist's life. The treater should acknowledge the patient would be missed but her life would continue as usual. Clients at high suicide risk should not be given lethal drugs and reassessed for the degree or measure of succeeding. Next we have:

Modifications of Psychotherapy with BPD

(Gabbard, The Menninger Project) [1] in light of new trauma data.

Aggression is understood in terms of an infantile self, rightly full of rage at parents.

Therapist must established a sense of safety for the patient.

Therapist needs to acknowledge and empathize with the patient's experience of being victimized (a very helpful validating strategy).

The patient's anger and manipulative behaviors need to be reframed as understandable, given the patient's early life experience (creates countertransference).

The therapeutic alliance in patients with BPD was correlated with the therapist interventions.

The client with early trauma, transference interpretation of the patient's aggression caused the alliance to deteriorate because the client experienced it as a lack of recognition that real tormentors were involved.

Empathic validation and affirmation of the client's perception improved the alliance.

Rightly Full of Rage at Parents

Given what borderlines have been though, they harbor anger, unable to contain it, they seek the all good object that they cannot destroy. Therapy should teach them emotional deregulation management.

Safety for the Patient

Boundaries must be established with clear consequences (Gabbard) [1]. The borderline incessantly will test limits hoping unconsciously to find immoveable lines of demarcation. It should be understood if the client needs evaluation and poses a danger to herself, the decision for hospitalization will be made by the emergency doctor. This modality will lift the responsibility from the treater and placing it in the hands of others, an applicable therapeutic measure to prevent manipulation or power struggles. Using this agency, a treater will impede countertransference feelings arising out of guilt. This is not to imply that all suicide ideation is borderline pathology, it could very well be a dysthymia depression advancing to major depression.

Interpretation of the Patient's Aggression

In other words, if the treater rejects the projected anger and interprets that the patient has wrongfully directed the anger toward the treater, then this will usually backfire since the client will feel that the treater has minimized his trauma.

Acknowledge and Empathize with the Patient's Experience

Typically, the borderline's past is riddled with chaotic battlefields of abuse and neglect amalgamated with an invalidating environment. The treater would do well not to re-victimize the client by continuing the act of the invalidating authoritarian. Survivors have a desire to be seen, heard and believed.

Manipulative Behaviors

Manipulative behaviors should be analyzed and dealt with according. On the other hand, what may look like manipulation to the treater may very well be the unconscious pathological signature of the borderline. Suppose for a moment (Linehan) [3], that a catastrophic earthquake nearly leveled a major city. The police, fireman and emergency crews are severely taxed. No one is able to help you. Trapped in the rubble within a small opening your child you love most in the world cries for help. The opening is too small for you to crawl through; if only she could move a couple of feet. You find a stick hoping that she is able to grasp it, but to no avail. Time is of the essence. Crews are asking people to clear the area. At any moment an aftershock is likely happen. The child is crying. She can't move because every bone in her body is broken! Do you suppose that she is manipulating you or just being difficult? Are you thinking that she will get out when she is ready? What would you do? Cheerlead, yell, plead, sweet-talk, suggest, threaten, distract and direct!

Therapeutic Alliance

Psychotherapy will not progress if the treater and client are at odds with each other. The treater should declare an armistice and construct common goals with the alliance of the client. A self proclaimed perennial omnipotent treater will find them self working with an severely un-pliable patient, which of course circumvents improvement.

Clinical Manifestations of Splitting in Adults

Alternating expression of contradictory behaviors.

Selected lack of impulse control.

The compartmentalization of individuals into, "all good" & "all bad" camps.

A coexistence of contradictory of self-representations that alternate with one another.

Alternating Expression

Part of a borderlines symptomatology is alternate expression. One moment the client will idealize a person and then completely devaluate them the next. They can experience severe mood shifts from high elation to despairingly low valleys. It's no wonder they often think they are losing their mind (Kreisman) [4].

References:

1. Integrated Treatment of Borderline Personality Disorder - Glen O. Gabbard, M. D. - Video Lecture / APA Series

2. Diagnostic and Statistical Manual of Mental Disorders DSM-IV-TR - American Psychiatric Association (APA)

3. Cognitive-Behavioral Treatment of Borderline Personality Disorder - Linehan

4. I Hate You, Don't Leave Me - Jerold Kreisman, M.D., Hal Straus

Into the Mind of the Borderline

Written by Kathi Stringer

Helpful note from a resistive patient with borderline personality disorder:

Help me when I deserve it the least. Help me in the face of my rage. It is easy to help me when I am the well behaved, the good-natured patient, but anyone without skill can treat me well when I am this way. I need your skills, your help when I am at my worst so that I can understand and identify something better than myself. You may have to show me over and over again that I have value and that my rage will not destroy you, because I learn these things slowly and my old ways are everywhere I look, they are in my thoughts and feelings. These thoughts and feelings feel like they will destroy me so I put them in you, because I hope you are stronger then I am.

So please don't be angry with me for putting these terrible feelings into you, and I hope that maybe you can do something with them because I don't know how or I need you to show me how with your actions so that I can identify with you. I try to understand your words but sometimes your words can't reach me because my emotions are asleep when you are talking but when my emotions are awake and disturb me, they are working in partnership with you, even if just a little.

So thank you for accepting and holding these terrible parts of myself and then letting me take them back after you have made them softer, easier to tolerate. Thank you for helping me when I least deserve it.

The above is straight from the mind of an individual with borderline personality disorder. *It incorporates object relations theory of the "container and the contained" and the "three levers of projective identification" to provide insight to help modify the closed internal objects of the client...i.e...take someone thing bad and exchange it for something better provided by the treater.*

The Childish BPD Adult

Written by Kathi Stringer

Talk to me as an adult and I will pretend to be exactly that. I pretend to be an adult to win as any child will do. When I pretend to be an adult, I am not in touch with my feelings or my core sense of self. It is like putting on a costume that is not mine but I can play the role. Because like a child, it is only play. It amazes me sometimes how well I can play the roles and fool others. If you try to reach me as an adult, you will have only air in your hands, a façade, a pretend element of what I am not. But if you can see, truly see beyond the adult toy masque, and see the child who operates all the adult mechanisms, then you see that which can be reached. If you talk to the pretend adult, then you will get pretend answers and behavior. But if you talk to the child, that which is I, then I can respond. This is my secret and for a long time even I didn't know this secret. It's hard to be a child in a grown up world. It's a feeling of being lost. It's sad sometimes because when I see other children they don't look lost. They have parents, structure and guidelines. This helped them grow and form into an adult. They went through the maze and arrived at the other end. It was a maze I have never had the opportunity to enter. What is structure? I remember at 6 being on the other side of town in the blackness of the night. No one cared where I was. What are parents? I can't ever remember being loved, rocked, cuddled or held. I have no memory traces of this. What are guidelines? I had none and made them up as I went along in life. I'm afraid my guidelines are not very stable since I didn't have a measuring stick that was constant in my life. Is it any wonder that I am still a lost child that is pretending to be an adult?

Engulfment of the Void

This is an example of how the child was reached. When Peggy and Dr. Witkowski highly recommended that I take medications but the choice was mine, I felt lost without structure. They were talking to what they thought was the adult part of me and since that part doesn't exist, I was not responding. It was too much of an adult choice and since I hated being anything like an adult I would not take part in that function, which involved making a choice. But when Dr. Witkowski talked to the child, and made the choice for the child - take the medication - the message went through all the vault doors and reached me. It's hard to explain the warmth and security when I am truly recognized for who I really am. For a moment I felt like I existed, that I was protected and had value. For a moment the abyss inside of me was gone. I felt contained and within some sort of nurturing structure. To those who grew up with parenting, this must seem like a puzzle to them because they yearned for the day they could break free from this binding parental structure. Yet, to never have it left me with undefined boundaries and a sense of being scattered and a loss of identity (Engulfment of the Void). So while making a choice represents freedom for some, for me it represents painful neglect of a child that had too many choices because nobody cared.

The Emotional Child - PTSD & Borderline Personality Disorder

Written by Kathi Stringer 2/6/04

I am emotional child, with a machine for a brain that won't turn off. The machine overtakes all matters of life, a distraction. The machine shifts into overdrive to evade, avoidance of self. Without the machine, the emotional child, hence `the child', would be lost without any delineated boundaries for containment. The machine provides the only known sense of object constancy, and even at that, it is a hologram. What remains without the machine is the abyss. The starving child that is lost in rapprochement, in endless reenactment, to secure a renewed experience from a failed situation.

Can I love as an adult? I suppose the machine can intellectually fabricate what may appear as the love from an adult. However, it is pretend, an act, an emulation from knowledge. I love as an emotional child, meaning, I love in a child vs. parental dynamic. This creates conflict between the machine and the child. The machine wants to be in control, to monitor the milieu, to prevent abuse, neglect and hurt. The child wants nothing to do with this role. The child wants to surrender, trust, and absorb the innocent essence of unconditional love. The machine and the child are hopelessly caught into developmental rapprochement, nomads land. The push-pull. The machine-child. The run, I test you, if you catch me, you love me, care for me. You miss, I look into my crystal ball, maybe you don't really love me. The machine builds walls, runs and plots a defense, all the while the child is screaming to be rescued from the machine. The machine is skilled, gifted, and prepared. The child is small, helpless, and insecure. If you talk to me as an adult, you are communicating with syntax formulas that are highly efficient. It is not real, but a carefully constructed defense operating out of insecurity. This creates problems. The child needs affection and trust when insecure. However, the machine intervenes and crystallizes a cellular matrix that takes control, because when the child is insecure, the machine is more defensive. When the child needs security the most, the machine starves it.

The Treater Blinks!

Written by Kathi Stringer

Working with Clients That Have
Borderline Personality Disorder

The Holding Environment

During the formation process of the therapeutic alliance a dual interview is taking place. The treater is gathering intake information to assess the symptomlogy of the client. The client however is looking for clues to determine the strengths and weaknesses of the treater. A client's unconscious preverbal structure may be inquiring whether or not the holding environment is defective.

Winnicott who coined the term '*holding environment*' felt it didn't need to be perfect but 'good enough'. He felt the failures of the holding environment would help adjust and acclimate the client to the difficulties encountered in reality.

Too Much, Too Soon

The traumatized and resistant client usually has an acute ability to size up the container that resides in the treater. If the treater's container presents itself as defective, clients may more then likely withhold information and unconsciously resist disclosure. A client may sense 'vibes' that to disclose sensitive material may be met with rejection. These 'vibes' may take the appearance that the treater is not qualified to contain the formless identity of the client's interpersonal dimensions.

Capitalize on Effective Defenses

It is not uncommon for some treaters to capitalize on the developed defenses of the false self that have enabled the client to function and meet the demands of their environment. However, the false self presents a problem when the client wakes up one day and asks, "Who am I? Have I simply been a pretender all along?"

When left with the haunting questions that one is a pretender, then the next line of thought may lead the client directly into the abyss, or as the DSM equates as 'emptiness'. Which brings us back to the fear of the defective container that resides in the treater.

In the early development of the therapeutic alliance, the client's distorted, formless and fragmented identity searches for a consistent and delineated personality structure in the treater. Hopefully the treater can present as the constant object and as an available template from which the client may investigate and examine their feelings without fear of overwhelming the treater.

A Protective Mistake

A novice treater may error on the side of caution hoping to protect the client and say something like this, "Perhaps these feelings are too painful for you, and perhaps it may be in your best interest to stop treatment." The treater in the client's mind has 'blinked' meaning that the holding environment is defective and cannot contain the painful organizations that dwell within the client. The client is back-handedly validated that the false self is healthier then the tormented true self that yearns for acceptance, nurturing and empathy. This suggestion from the treater may circumvent the true self back into the abyss under the guise of keeping the more sophisticated defenses intact. A gain of this type is nothing but smoke and mirrors that dilutes motivation for further investigation and the client may be left with the impulsive recoil to go along with the treater's suggestion and 'quit'.

You're Right, I Quit.

The client may quit out of hatred because the treater has exposed the treater's defected container. The disappointed client is now in a foolish and humiliated light that was induced by the sham of hope. After all, it was suggested by the treater that the true self could be written off and barred in favor of more useful and adaptive false self. The whole scenario may come off as being used again, "You don't like me, only who I am able to pretend to be."

The Alternative

In the genesis of the new holding environment, a highly defended client must be able to internalize that an alternate supportive structure from the treater can maintain some measure of protection. This invites the client to view the world without the safety of the armored false self. It stands to reason, before one can venture out into a dangerous situation, the partner must provide a sense of protection. Akin to the ole western movies, that when one makes a break for it, the other will provide cover.

Basically, when a traumatized client's pain presents as 'non-adaptive', remember…

Don't Blink and Cover!

I Win!

At the end of my therapy session, I looked at the clock and said, "I win!" and my treater admitted it was true, that I had won. Meaning that for the last hour I had managed to keep her away from my feelings under the cloak of intellectual rotations. Her quick response on my way out enquired as to why winning was so important to me. I offered that in winning, maybe I really lost? In a single moment, she had delivered the ball back in my court. I left.

What did I mean by, "I win?" It was time to mull it over because in the real sense of 'winning' I don't think I won anything. The phrase certainly did seem like a puzzle. At the same time I was engaged at holding true to my intellectual stance. Then it became clear to me.

Winning to me meant to be successful. I was exactly that! I was successful at playing the role assigned to me as a child. One of the characterlogical parameters for this role required the ability to ignore and disregard my feelings. Not to do so was internalized as weak, and weak was to lose.

My impression as a child was that only the weak would cry and express vulnerability. And the strong? Strength was measured by the appearance of an inflexible stance or expressions of anger. Strength adapted the abilities to isolate and eradicate the pitiful whinnying of weakness that manifested as a desire of be loved, touched and held. Absurd! Such thoughts evoked shame. After all, there is shame in weakness. Sissies are weak.

To be strong is to have approval and divert attention away from weakness. Any suspicion that would invite exanimation that would reveal the cry of the all-encompassing longing to be swallowed up in love and nurturing must be thwarted, sidetracked and eliminated. Winning approval in this distorted reality meant to deprive myself of the healthy narcissistic needs of a child to be the center of parental love.

I have played my assigned role successfully, meaning, I have won. Yet how strange, the prize was destroyed in the mechanics that are intrinsic of the game.

The prize was to be loved and held as a diminutive being that is now lost in the past. As the winner, I collect a deceptive and distorted victory, and the swindle escapes accountability.

Now, it is a time for restructuring, reframing, and reorganizing. As a developmentally fixated child, my true-self, I don't know how. I am a rock. I am an island.

Now the ball is back in her court.

What Kind of Therapy is Best for You?

Written by Kathi Stringer

Before making that phone call for a therapist, there are a couple of things to consider, the type of therapy and the expense. We'll go over each and their approaches so that you can judge what may be best for you. Also, these suggestions are designed for borderline personality disorder as the principal diagnosis.

The two main therapeutic treatments for borderline personality disorder are Dialectical Behavior Therapy (DBT) and Psychodynamic Psychotherapy.

Dialectical Behavior Therapy (DBT)

DBT has the advantage since empirical evidence lends proof it is the most successful for treating borderline personality disorder. The focus on DBT is acceptance vs. change. The therapists are trained to help you with your 'thinking' process for problem solving in conjunction with getting validation. The treatment works on the postulation that borderline behavior stems from poor emotional regulation and slow return to baseline once aroused. DBT is similar to cognitive behavior therapy with added features. Figure on once weekly group sessions and well as once weekly individual sessions along with homework assignments.

If you need firm structure, then this may be your best choice.

Psychodynamic Psychotherapy

This therapy is more flexible and not as rigged as DBT and it works around several components, which are exploration, interpretation, confrontation, clarification and support. The therapist gives special attention to the 'therapist and client relationship' looking for clues from the behavior a client brings into the office. Problems in the here-and-now are addressed for immediate action and afterward unresolved issues from the past are examined. Supportive measures of validation, empathy, listening, and offering comfort are offered to help nurture the client. Psychodynamic psychotherapy has the advantage of helping the client with insight by bringing the unconscious into the conscious where it can be examined and reworked. When this happens the therapist is able to offer something more attractive for the client.

Psychodynamic Psychotherapy has the advantage of the 'Parent and Child' dyad for those clients that suffer from separation and loss from early childhood.

Crazy Therapies

As with any therapy, be careful of what you are getting yourself into. There are just about as many therapies out there as there are therapists. For an in depth look at how crazy some of them can get, this book would be a good read, "Crazy Therapies."

References:

1. Cognitive-Behavioral Treatment of Borderline Personality Disorder [Book Link]
2. Skills Training Manual for Treating Borderline Personality Disorder [Book Link]
3. Psychiatric Annals, June 2002
4. Harvard Letter, March 2002
5. Crazy Therapies

Manipulation and the Borderline Personality Disorder

Written by Kathi Stringer

What exactly is manipulation, and are individuals with borderline personality disorder capable of this sort of exploitation?

This area of discussion is thought provoking and has been tossed around quite a bit. Usually the prominent mental health professionals agree that a person with borderline personality disorder is a very poor manipulator (Gabbard, Linehan, Mason and Iowa model). They are indeed so pitiable at management of their behaviors that it often lands them into trouble. For this paper it will be useful to separate cognition from behavior to isolate manipulation.

Cognition

Manipulation is defined as a deliberate thought process. Not behavior, but thought. A cognitive, shrewd, artful....planning, setting into motion a plan, an idea and make that idea a reality. Scientists manipulate genes, lab rats and additional parameters, skillfully and deliberately. Not as a reflex. When the mind is skillfully forming specific algorithmic (step-by-step) instructions, then we can call this manipulation.

Reactive Behavior

Manipulation is a response, not a reaction. Knee-jerk is a reaction. Again, we go to the definition of the word. Manipulation is defined as a thought process, not a behavior process. Behavior is only the product. This product of reaction, a sort of pseudo-manipulation is usually activated when an individual with borderline personality perceives impending annihilation, disaster and abandonment. This hypersensitivity may stir up tremendous anxiety and helplessness.

Helplessness

Most people with a borderline personality have not successfully moved though their early developmental stages and are fixated usually around 2 to 4 years of age. Impulsivity is a prominent behavior that is often misinterpreted as manipulation. A person with borderline personality may experience anxiety as helplessness since she cannot equate her notions to an adult on an equal level. As one person living with an individual with borderline personality stated,

"I suspect that the BP at this point is in maddening, excruciating emotional pain and confusion."

Her take on this portrays helplessness especially well since time becomes narrowed and pressured giving a sense of urgency to resolve the pain. This sets into motion a reactive reflex (pseudo-manipulation) to ward off anxiety with often-destructive consequences. These destructive measures amount to job loss or relationship failure due to poor strategies to resolve antithetical troubles, hardly an artful and shrewd manipulation of a mastermind.

Barry Kiehn and Michaela Swales Stated:

"Linehan has a particular dislike for the word "manipulative" as commonly applied to these patients [borderline]. She points out that this implies that they are skilled at managing other people when it is precisely the opposite that is true. Also the fact that the therapist may feel manipulated does not necessarily imply that this was the intention of the patient. It is more probable that the patient did not have the skills to deal with the situation more effectively."

The Iowa model

University of Iowa Department of Psychiatry; The STEPPS Group Treatment Program for Borderline Personality Disorder stated:
"Rather than viewing themselves [individuals with borderline personality disorder] as someone who is attempting to manipulate, is attention-seeking, or is sabotaging treatment, the trainees [individuals with borderline personality disorder] learn to view themselves as driven by the disorder to seek relief from a painful illness through desperate behaviors which are reinforced by negative and distorted thinking."

An individual with borderline personality has the ability to manipulate, however; it is not the principal process of artful cognition that leads to borderline-style behavior. If we are going to use the term 'behavior' then it is more parallel to defensive behavior. Most of the time a borderline adapts to defensive behavior rather then manipulative behavior. There is an immense differentiation between primitive borderline defense mechanisms and skillful manipulation, the product of each, which is behavior.

Co-morbid Axis II diagnosis

What comes to mind is the Narcissist who co-opts others to carry out her functions. For example the narcissist doesn't have the ability to feel empathy for others, and uses others as her narcissist supply, needing constant approval, strokes and identity assurance. The narcissist personality is not what society assumes, having a 'big ego, just the opposite, they use the ego (executive of the self) of others because they are truly empty. Once these needs are not getting met any longer, the narcissist personality will easily dump the target and move onto the next. Quite different from the borderline personality, a narcissist personality is extremely good at manipulating, and their defensives are more advanced then the borderline personality.

It is helpful to consider that often times a person that has borderline personality is a 'mixed bag' since comorbidity traits in patients with borderline personality disorder is high. However if borderline personality disorder is the principle personality structure, chances are they are poor manipulators.

Treatment Team Awareness

Multidisciplinary staff and treaters would jeopardize the therapeutic alliance if they did not have a clear understanding of the borderline personality defenses. This is why countertransference management is important. Borderlines can make a treater's veins budge out of the side of their necks, in a snap. As one treater recommended, "remove the hook." Much easier said then done, it takes practice. Once a treatment team realizes that a borderline personality reacts, rather then the assumed fraudulent observation of manipulation, a strong therapeutic alliance is easier to construct since manipulation engenders hatred from the professional community.

Conclusion

Manipulation is a deliberate and artful thought process, which is not a common trait found in the borderline personality. The borderline personality defense is closer a Reactive Defense Mechanism that operates as a knee-jerk retort flung into motion from a low threshold of impulsivity. Identifying the difference between manipulation and reaction to painful stimuli can help ameliorate the therapeutic stance.

References:

1. Cognitive-Behavioral Treatment of Borderline Personality Disorder - M. Linehan
2. Skills Training Manual for Treating Borderline Personality Disorder - M. Linehan
3. The Iowa model http://www.vh.org/Patients/IHB/Psych/Treatment/stepps.html
4. Barry Kiehn and Michaela Swales at http://www.priory.com/dbt.htm

The Responsibility of Change and the Individual with Borderline Personality Disorder

Written by Kathi Stringer

Change. It is a word that provokes anxiety in some of the healthiest clients. But to a person with borderline personality disorder (borderline) it can be terrifying. Imagine having a shaky sense of identity, and even that which is known, is about ready to be annihilated though the process of change. Change doesn't go over well with a borderline that craves object constancy, a developmental level skipped over in childhood, because it seems they are now threaten with the aspect of giving up that which is familiar and compulsive for the apparent, aggressive dynamic of change.

The Roadways of Change

In metropolitan cities traffic usually runs smoother when using two-lane roads. It is the one-way streets that can get confusing. Imagine a city with only one-way streets and trying to navigate your way around. It seems understandable a two-lane street would be more efficient by providing a greater access for delivery. It is with this paper I hope to remind the treater that there are <u>Two Executive Deliveries for Change.</u>

(1) Client-Induced Change

Goals are often established with the onset of therapy built on the foundation that the client needs to change. Simply, it's not what happens to the client but rather how a client reacts to the event. Cognitive behavioral treaters usually approach change from examining the client's cognitive structures and will then suggest modification in certain identified areas to address a client's emotional anxiety to stimuli (Linehan-DBT). However, most Cognitive Behavioral Therapy (CBT) offers only a single technique for change and referred to as 'Client-induced' since it places the full weight of change onto the client. Client-induced change can be extremely frustrating for the client since regression and failures are viewed as the client's responsibility... i.e. "you choose to feel this way." The rest of this paper will now focus on the second avenue for change.

(2) Treater-Induced Change

At the opposite end of the continuum is a method for change referred to as 'Treater-induced '. Treater-induced modus operandi centers on the artful skills of the treater as an agent of psychodynamic psychotherapy (Gabbard). Actively, it is the treaters' holding environment and detoxification of the projected objects (anger in this example) that will bring about change in the client. Treater-induced because the treater is offering to the client material that was projected onto the treater that has been contained and modified (changed by the treater) and is now more manageable for the client and available for assimilation into the client's closed internal system. (see more on introjective identification)

Analogy of the Blacksmith

The blacksmith must first heat the material before it can skillfully be reworked into a precious measurement of success. If the blacksmith were to attempt to shape cold metal his efforts would be a consuming and daunting process. In other words a bit of heat helps in the reshaping development. Using a procedure of gently challenging (triggering) the client, the work then becomes warm and provides access for the treater to rework and modify the closed internal system of the client.

When to Hold and When to Fold

As any successful poker player will tell you, winning the game depends on the strategy. How to play the hand depends on the strength of the cards. Similar to poker the degree of success from therapy would depend on when to use confrontation and when to use supportive measures. For example, if a treater triggers a client using confrontation and then the client's emotions become intolerable, the client may threaten to duck out of therapy, which at this time the apparent move would be to fold and use a supportive stance.

Analogy of Gently Stirring the Pot

If a treater finds themselves wrapped around a client's finger, with sessions that are dull, flat and unproductive, then the reason is more then likely the treater is failing to stir the pot. The unresolved conflicts of the client are usually lying at the bottom of the pot in the form of sludge. By stirring the pot a treater can see what comes up so that it may be identified and reworked. I would recommend using a wooden ladle, a metaphor for ego-detachment and countertransference management to protect the treater's hands from getting burned.

Containment for Change

As one treater said, 'this anger you are projecting is yours and not mine", to which the client replied, "can you think of anything better to do with it?" This is what separates the amateurs from the professionals. A professional is able to, contain, metabolize, detoxify and modify the projected object (anger) and then offer a more manageable form to the client, a second avenue for change (Bion).

Effective Treatment in the Region of Rejection

I want to shift gears for a moment and touch on the issue of rejection. It stands to reason the client needs a safe place to project their anger in the presence of the all-good-object and will not be excommunicated from the family relationship of the patient-therapist dyad. Some treaters because of their own unresolved conflicts place counterproductive boundaries on the therapeutic relationship. Some are unable to contain the projected bad object (anger) of the client and threaten to ban the client from the practice. For the individual with borderline personality disorder, they may respond in much the same way an angry child would from being banned from the family relationship. It could have a devastating effect. A threat like this runs the risk of validating the unconscious belief that 'I am not lovable and I can destroy the all-good-object" and rejection is always just around the corner. For a borderline personality with separation and abandonment issues, this may fixate therapy because no matter what the re-enactment, rejection is the precarious dreaded monster. It is advisable to be prudent when setting the execution boundary to mitigate rejection fears.

Summary

Working with the borderline personality is a challenge. It is helpful when we are able to identify two avenues for change, client-induced and treater-induced. Client-induced change maximizes the cognitive behavioral techniques, while treater-induced change is a skillful and artful technique of modifying the client's internal closed objects. Client-induced change is usually more effective and available to the client when the client is challenged (triggered).

Section ii

"Letters & Questions

about

Borderline Personality Disorder "

Disclosing Borderline Personality Disorder to an Undiagnosed Spouse

Written by Kathi Stringer
July 29, 2003

> This is great advice - it's informative and the communication ideas are very helpful - Cristina Cabrera, M.A.
> Interpersonal Communication

Question:

Should a person be told they have borderline personality disorder? My wife is unaware she is a BP. The advice I had from the Psychologist is that it would not be helpful for my wife to know she is a BP and in fact it might be damaging. I find it difficult to withhold information as having been marriage 42 years I have always operated on sharing our lives in all ways. I can go on withholding this information if it is the wisest path to follow.

At different times I have tried to open the subject but there is always a reaction of hostility. I have attached a note I gave her in the hopes it would open the doorway to my being able to discuss the matter. It definitely got the thumbs down and only started a hostile reaction. The general reaction is to tell me I need fixing and that she is all right. Unfortunately over the years I have approached a number of professional people (who did not understand borderline personality disorder) and she subsequently came along. I think she is now at the stage of professional burnout after so much unhelpful information.

I have approached our local psychiatric unit and they have a program running to assist BP. It seems that it would be very helpful to her, but unless she knows she is a BP and approaches them they cannot help.

I believe that knowledge is power and it seems to me that if you know all that facts about yourself that you are in the best position to make decisions.

Have you any thoughts on this matter, as I would like your opinion. I realize it's a knotty question.

Answer:

The Undiagnosed Insult

There is quite a bit of information against disclosing a possible diagnosis of borderline personality disorder (BPD) to those we love and care about….and for good reason. The phrase "personality disorder" comes across as an insult, even in the kindest delivery. For example, imagine if you felt there was nothing wrong with your intelligence and someone empathetically tried to convince that you were in denial and that you are actually severely retarded. How would that go over? Perhaps you may recoil and shout, "I'm not stupid, you are the stupid one!" Then of course, things get escalated from there and any therapeutic window for discussion is now highly defended.

Identity Expansion

There is a second reason, however that may keep a treater from disclosing a diagnosis. Lets say for example through discussion with the treater it is agreed the client meets the minimum of 5 of the 9 symptoms for Borderline Personality Disorder [1]. Now lets say the client suffers from confusion and is lacking identity. Now we have a troubled client that is relived to meet the newly official diagnostic criteria to open a pathway toward individuality (upgrades to identity). Of course the client is excited to learn more about herself and studies all of the symptoms for a diagnosis of borderline personality disorder. Through research the client finds there are 4 more symptoms that she has managed to keep 'in check' but now realizes she has some latitude, a more extensive range to express her newly discovered identity. It is as though she has received a license to be complete, however maladaptive that may be. The reasoning maybe, "An maladaptive identity is better then no identity at all." Now we have a treater that is frustrated with the extra symptoms that the client had previously been able to manage. So now what? Lets look at a few other items first and find out what a 'disordered' diagnosis amounts too.

The DSM-IV-TR

The DSM-IV is a dialogistic manual to aid treaters to formulate a diagnosis [1]. The DSM-IV views personality problems as 'disorders.' Therefore, it may be helpful to take a closer look at the DSM and understand how 'disorders' are rated.

The DSM-IV splits up a comprehensive diagnosis into five different categories referred to as "Axis". Axis One is basically reserved for disorders that are treated with the 'medical model' such as Bipolar, Schizophrenia and Schizoaffective. Axis Two is reserved for the personality disordered such as NPD and borderline personality disorder. The primary difference between Axis One and Axis Two equates to the 'medical model' vs. 'developmental model.' In other words, Axis one in more likely to be treated primarily with medication, and Axis Two with talk therapy as a way to work though the arrested developments. (Note: Mental Retardation is also on Axis Two) Axis Three relates to prior or ongoing physical problems such as cancer, surgery or physical limitations. Axis Four relates to environmental or situational problems that may be giving rise to some of the symptoms. Axis

Five (GAF) relates to the Global Functioning Scale that is rated from 0 to 100. Zero would be suicide and 100 would be perfect functioning.

A DSM-IV Diagnosis goes something like this:

Axis 1: Depression NOS [Not otherwise specified], rule out Bipolar

Axis 2: Borderline Personality Disorder, Severe

Axis 3: Lacerations of the wrist and diabetic

Axis 4: Relationship problems, job loss and legal problems

Axis 5: 10 (suicidal, liable, unpredictable and confused)

When it comes to care planning a doctor is required to make a diagnosis on each axis along with the driving symptoms.

Disorder vs. Organization

The word 'disorder' immediately suggests a defect. There are some grassroots' organizations and individuals that are peeved at the notion of being labeled as disordered, and for good reason, because in some cases at the risk of annihilation they created these psychological structures to help them survive an abusive childhood. It comes off as a double negative. First, the individual is beat up in childhood and second, they are beat up again as being labeled disordered.

Otto Kernberg, a proliferated writer, theorist, and treater is a distinguished expert on borderline personality disorder. However, Kernberg refers to borderline personality disorder as "Borderline Personality Organization" [3],[4] which seems to relive the stigma somewhat, and recognize the personality as an adaptive organization at the time when higher levels of defensives were not yet constructed within the mind. Kernberg recognized that 'borderline organization' is an arrested developmental phenomenon that remained ridged in the personality because abuse or neglect road blocked expansion to age appropriate adaptive defensives.

Symptomology

Personally, I think I would rather be identified as relating to others with a certain 'personality organization' instead of 'personality disorder.' The mitigated descriptive use of 'organization' is helpful to invite self-examination of 'symptoms' rather then disorder – defect. The treater and the client have a greater advantage toward treatment if collaboration is focused on the acute symptoms rather then the pigeonhole disorder.

Treatment Considerations

Now lets move on toward disclosure of 'personality organization' to a loved one to facilitate treatment. Frankly, an accusation of an 'undiagnosed' personally disorder toward a loved one, no matter how well intended can stir up a tit-for-tat problem. Before proceeding we need to consider a few things first.

- Have these symptoms always existed before a commitment to marriage?
- Have the symptoms escalated over time during the marriage?
- How likely is it that your spouse will accept the idea of treatment for their symptoms?
- How important is the idea of having peace in your life?
- Are you willing to make sacrifices to have a more rewarding life?

These are important questions, because when it comes down to it, you cannot help anyone if they are not willing to accept that help (Stringer) [4]. If your spouse gets into treatment, that is one thing, but refusal begs for another question to be asked of yourself. "Can I continue in this relationship the way things are going?"

To help answer this question, consider that all relationships are 'value-for-value.' Are you getting enough of what you need to stay in the relationship? If not, consider your option of leaving. If you decide to stay in the relationship, ask yourself what you are receiving emotionally or physically, and is it worth the trade-off?

Changing A Person

Often co-dependent couples are disillusioned with romantic love and there is a sense of "I can fix her, and change her, and make her whole" and on the flip side "he can save me, provide for me, and nurture me, and make me whole." Then later down the road it dawns on the fixer that he is not able to fix or change his spouse. It was assumed by the fixer that once married and his gift of 'fixing' were engaged, the partner would heal and everything would be hunky-dory. Instead things may have gotten worse because the spouse cannot get fixed enough and will up the stakes to bring on more of an urgency to be fixed. So, things have indeed changed, but for the worse because the needy became more needy and burnout is just over the horizon. In essence, relationships are practically doom for failure if one or both partners are not happy at the point of marriage and are expecting 'change.' Basically, a person 'marries' what they agreed to marry when they say, "I do."

Discussion Time

If you want to try and save the relationship, then set a time aside for discussion. Try it again. Make sure you toss the word "I" and use "Us - We - Our" to denote "we are in this together" For example, "Honey, I would like to spend some time with you and discuss something very important to us. Is there a time when we can do that?" Then later at that time "Thank you for making time for us, it is very important to me and I appreciate it." Then… "I am very concerned about 'our' relationship. We are having problems communicating and getting our needs met. I'm afraid if we don't get some outside coaching soon, we may not be able to survive our marriage." Expand on this as much as you like, but make it about 'we' and it will increase your chances of getting treatment going. Accusatory statements such as 'you made me' or 'you did it' or 'it's not my fault' will create setbacks and a defensive stance. Save those problems for your treater.

In Treatment

Once treatment has begun, begin with sessions together and also apart to express concerns. As things move along, hopefully the individual that needs the treatment the most can receive it and the other individual can decrease treatment or discontinue all together. Once in treatment the treater can make judgment calls as to the timely revelation of the full Axis workup for the client, whereby taking you off the hook.

Treatment Refusal

Now we are back to the phrase "value-for-value.' Are you willing to live with a person that refuses to seek treatment? Do you think that getting treatment for yourself can help you continue to live with your spouse, and enhance your chances for happiness? I would suggest that you try it, or continue the relationship as usual, or dissolve the relationship.

These are hard choices for sure but the problem will not go away, only the remainder of your time on this earth toward a chance for happiness will go away. Something to think about.

***Summery*:**

- A suggestion of borderline personality can come off as an insult.
- A diagnosis of Borderline Personality Disorder can provide an identity for those lost in emptiness and therefore may increase the symptoms.
- A diagnosis toward care planning is categorized in 5 Axis'.
- Kernberg's borderline organization is less demeaning then borderline disorder.
- Addressing symptoms has its advantages for getting a person into treatment rather than the tit-for-tat insult of 'personality defect.'
- Consider the value-for-value to remain in the relationship.
- It is not fair to expect a person to change after marriage.
- Setup a time for discussion
- Enter treatment as 'We' rather than the accusatory 'you' to get things moving along.
- Consider options if treatment is refused.

***References*:**

Diagnostic and Statistical Manual of Mental Disorders DSM-IV-TR - American Psychiatric Association (APA)
[Book Link]
Severe Personality Disorders - Otto F. Kernberg
[Book Link]
Borderline Conditions and Pathological Narcissism - Otto F. Kernberg
[Book Link]
Breaking Free from Co-dependence - Kathi Stringer
[Page Link]

Questions From Individuals with BPD

Written by Kathi Stringer

- Part 1: Considering Leaving a DBT Program
- Part 2: Professional crossed Boundaries

Considering Leaving a DBT Program 11/10/02

***Question*:** I have been in a DBT program for 20 weeks due to my intense worshipping to a punishing God that I grew up with. The staff and I have had several misunderstandings. It is almost my time to leave the program and I feel that I am not ready; however, because the past 20 weeks I have been what I call myself is a "high maintenance" client and I do have severe and complex PTSD. I want to ask for the end of Dec. to be the end of my program. I feel as though the staff would rather just get rid of me, I haven't made much progress and that I am a failure (tears).

***Answer*:** With severe BPD, 20 weeks of DBT is only a blink of time. It takes years in most cases to treat borderline personality disorder. Of course there will be misunderstandings along the way. We are talking about borderline personality disorder personalities here. If you are not ready, then you are not ready. You know yourself better then the treaters working with you.

As for being a 'high maintenance' client, many borderline personalities are. In that realm, you are normal. And, many treaters believe that PTSD and borderline personality disorder have much in common. PTSD comes from a stance of pro survival and BPD is looked at as more manipulative, which in most cases is false.

When considering leaving the program, think back if your treaters are frustrated or irritated. It is a normal response for a treater to become frustrated at times when goals are not reached. However, irritation comes from the wish that a client would disappear, which of course can stir rejection and abandonment issues in the client. Think about this and sort out the two. In addition, if a treater is truly a professional, they will encourage you to stay in the program, if not, then it would be wise to consider whether or not you are truly dealing with a professional.

I can see that you are very depressed. When all your thoughts seem heavy and close in on you, try to remember that persistence will always win out.

In other words, no matter your thoughts, keep trying, and one day you WILL get there.

Professional crossed Boundaries Nov 04 2002

Question: I'm a 47-yrar-old female with an M.S. Ed. Teaching 12 yrs. 2 grown daughters (w/degrees) and success. The Psychiatrist I've been seeing for 2 1/2 years started using terminology about 3 months ago about BPD without ever posing (?) for a diagnosis. I was never told a diagnosis from the beginning. From early on, he said we were friends. We've gone for coffee, wings, met him & his daughter at the bookstore. Several times I expressed upset at lack of confidentiality and he got annoyed with me. Everything has changed now. He yells at me really bad & when I've told him not to yell at me he says he will. Then he told me I crossed boundaries!!! Every time I try and repair our relationship he screams, " I'm not the one in therapy! This is NOT about ME!!"

Why does one part of my intuition tell me to leave and yet another part of me cries about him? He's 47 too and the head of a psychiatric floor of a hospital. I feel terrible. I feel worse than when I started therapy (because of a divorce after 28 yrs. of marriage. I know I have some tendencies of BPD, but can't they mimic PTSD? I was sexually, physically, and emotionally abused as a child. Please help me. I feel so frightened about being a BPD!

Answer: It appears this psychiatrist did not act professionally. He 'did' violate professional boundaries when mixing a casual relationship with professional therapeutic interventions.

For goal setting and care planning, he should have included you as to the information of your dx. After all, how can goals be set if one does not understand the symptoms?

Additionally, needless dependence/negative transference issues have risen because he allowed a relationship to develop outside of the office.

As for staying because he 'has the power to write things about you that aren't true", he has that power regardless if you decide to stay or leave. So this should not be an issue for deciding to continue (mis) treatment with him.

As for him using terms to sidetrack you, it is exactly that. At least it appears that way from what you have told me.

He 'screams' at you. This is poor countertransference management (Stringer) [3]. He is supposed to be the 'professional' and not you.

Last, it is ALWAYS sad to connect to a person that continues the abuse cycle. Based on your history with your family, it is repeating again through him via 'The Trauma Bond'. See more here:

The Trauma Bond (Ross) [1]
and here
The Victim-Rescuer-Perpetrator Triangle (Ross) [2]

This is all I can do, to advise. If it were me, I would leave. Now. Magical thinking is not going to repair anything.

Sorry you are going through so much. Take courage,
Kathi Stringer

Reply

Thank-you, Kathi for responding to my e-mails. I tell my students if they have an "uh-oh feeling" they should listen to it because nature gives us these instincts. I should follow my own advice no matter how sad I feel. Staying will only prolong the pain. I wish I didn't feel like it's all my fault. Thanks, again.

***References*:**

1. The Trauma Bond - Colin Ross M.D. - Edited / Kathi Stringer [Page Link]
2. The Victim-Rescuer-Perpetrator Triangle - Colin Ross M.D. [Page Link]
3. The Secret Language of the Psychotherapist - Kathi Stringer [Page Link]

Borderline Personality Disorder and Fragmentation

Written by Kathi Stringer

Question:
"Could he know what he was doing and that it was wrong? To me it was intentional and could have been prevented, not unintentionally created by a mental disorder."

Answer:
This maybe true. Just an after thought for consideration...

In some of the more severe individuals with bpd there is a complete fragmentation. It becomes really confusing since so many statements and behaviors appear to be contradictory. Believe it or not, some are unable to bridge the pathological process of opposing thoughts. Then what happens is the internal drama of the bpd is played out in reality. A person gets a taste of their internal confusion.

Some individuals do have a sense of an internal connection and this is helpful because it offers them a chance to tune-in to what is going on...to help bridge the internal compartmentalization. As if with practice an individual with bpd can observe and integrate these conflicting views. Some bpd's when severely emotionally disturbed have no avenue to make a connection of the self and what is going on inside them is the mirror of what is going on outside them. For example if a person is getting conflicting and opposite statements, this is exactly what is happening in the mind of a bpd. Pure conflict and comes off as irrational thought. What it really is, is thought that hasn't been combined and processed. Sort of what a person sees is Freud's Primary Process to rid disturbing impulses quickly in raw form, rather then the more integrated Secondary Process of reason in the developing ego.

I guess in a way, one side does know what they are doing and the other side doesn't have a clue. What an individual with bpd projects, is what is going on inside them. If it appears to look like confusion, opposite, conflicting and contrary from one statement to the next...then you can get an idea of the drama going within the individual.

Borderline Personality Disorder, Stress and Mood Swings

Written by Kathi Stringer

Question:

My friend is facing a lot of stress in his own life and has become even more moody and sometimes quite distant. Then he suddenly latches on again for reassurance. Is this typical behavior? The dark mood seems to be engulfing as the stress on him increases. He lashes out in anger and then regrets are expressed within a day or 2....

Answer:

The degree of apparent moodiness sometimes correlates with two operands, stress and the degree of poorly integrated internal objects. The more primitive and unintegrated the personality structure, the more confusing the behavior appears since it oscillates at times rapidly. The primary defense is splitting or primitive dissociation and becomes more pervasive as emotions rise leading to intense regression.

When triggered, TIME for most individuals with borderline personality disorder becomes narrowed or pressured. The focal point is acute giving rise to a sense that immediate action is necessary to ward off overwhelming anxieties. Since each internal object is associated with its own affect and lacks a global cohesiveness, then mood seems to change as rapidly as the individual with borderline personality disorder focuses on different external objects with analogous qualities. [1] Kernbreg stated, "Primitive transferences are rapidly mobilized, highly distorted, fragmented, and ephemeral. They reflect the patient's lack of a stable sense of self or significant others."

For example, under stress, repressed object representations (love or hate from the past) are reactivated and resurrected from the there-and-then with their accompanying affects (emotions) into the here-and-now. The old objects that are resurrected with the old emotions that go with them are 'transferred' onto another person. In reality, the old objects and affects are a distortion (belonging to a past event) but they are amplified in the transference. One may think, "I have awoken the monster within." Which sounds about right because without stress, it is far easier to manage what is real, with what is not real (the past). Under stress, the fragile system goes on the blink and everything gets lumped together, old material with new material. Since unintegrated objects have binding affects, the individual with borderline personality disorder experiences the situation as dynamically intense in the present as they had in the past because stress lowers the threshold of ego strength.

If it seems extremely confusing to the observer, imagine the confusion due to the inability to integrate thoughts into the secondary process of the executive ego in the borderline individual.

One of the primary goals of psychodynamic psychotherapy is to integrate the compartmentalized objects from a primitive fixation that is insufficiently integrated (part-objects) into a more advanced and continuous global object relations. Work moves to establish an observing ego so that one hand knows what the other hand is doing (thinking).

Why: Splitting, primitive dissociation, projecting part objects and representations, primitive transferences, and STRESS.

Solution: Development of an observing ego and integration of fragmented self into a more global object representation. Stress management.

Reference:

1. (1989) Psychodynamic Psychotherapy of the Borderline Patients / Kernberg, Selzer, Koenigsberg, Carr and Appelbaum.
[Book Link]

Questions About Therapy and Borderline Personality Disorder

by Kathi Stringer

Question

I wonder how to tell which type of treatment would be best for me, e.g.. Dialectical behavioral therapy, or schema therapy? Do you have an opinion on who benefits from which outpatient therapy? Is one clearly better than another?

Answer

I think the main thrust for fragmented individuals in outpatient therapy gives them structure. A sense of being contained while they can work on their problems.

Cognitive Behavior Therapy (CBT) is a good choice for most all dx's except BPD. CBT was tried on borderlines but it had somewhat of a negative effect at times. CBT has an invalidating component to the sensitive borderline. Dialectical Behavior Treatment (DBT) was created to include validation. "I accept you the way you are (validation) as long as you will commit to change." I know some treaters in group will square-off and confront an individual on their views, and those having BPD will stand their ground, may even be triggered into self-harm or some other impulsive act after group. Yet, CBT is better then nothing for those with BPD if they can understand the nature of CBT before going in and letting it get to them.

As you know, some treaters have an assortment of tricks to bring into group therapy. Medication, breathing, role-playing.... Some use David Burns material to identify feelings from reality. Thoughts are not actions..etc.

Question.

Thanks for your reply, especially the explanation about validation and CBT vs DBT. I wonder if you'd be willing to answer another question: My biggest relationship problem is with myself, because of an introject that sees me as bad and causes misery whenever I start to feel good about myself. What type of therapeutic approach is most likely to help me reduce this part of myself? Will it always be a part of me?

Answer:

This question is much more difficult. Before one can ameliorate a problem, one must understand it. There could be a Drama Triangle in process, (the victim, rescuer, persecutor rotation) or an unconscious wish for quasi-parental intervention, or resistance to relinquish that which is familiar known, or the damming ego-ideal as the relentless inner critic sabotaging your self-esteem.

You could research, learn, and study. However, this said, it is also going to take some extensive talk therapy. Knowing and understanding is usually not enough. You could have extensive knowledge of psych, yet the knowledge is only 'instructions' on how to get there, and getting there involves a process – teamwork. For example, I could build a fantastic ride at Disneyland, but that doesn't mean I could ever understand the feeling or thrill of the ride unless I got on it myself. See what I mean? Building, planning and designing is one facet of treatment/therapy, but experiencing it is all together another.

Lets say I'm in therapy. My treater is hitting on a nerve. I began to escalate. My emotions are coming up, and out. I am now in touch with that which was closed off, like molten lava in the center of the earth. Now, a CBT treater would typically confront me and may say something like, "This is your anger, I don't want it crammed down my throat." This comes off as invalidation, because my anger was amplified from unresolved material buried so down deep, that I have a hard time understanding it. I hear it as I don't have a right to that anger. Now Mr. CBT is confronting and intimidating me into stuffing it back down again where it will continue to stew. And, as Glen Gabbard M.D. stated, "This will usually backfire." However, a skillful treater will 'go with it' and see where the anger in the transference takes us as joint partnership looking for answers, that is to feel, and process, that which is buried, and cut-off. If done correctly, I may experience a wonderful cathartic release. It is in my opinion, tapping into that which is distant, and confusing, can give the most healing and transforming results.

Treatment can open many doors of the unknown, and like a broken puzzle, will hold a picture after all the pieces are looked at one-by-one and placed into canvas. As Vaknin Ph.D. explained, ***"It is an intricate and subtle dance of aggression ("bad object") and counter-aggression, neediness and rejection, attraction and repulsion, assignment of roles and their assumption, assimilation and denial, insight and cognitive distortions. It is a hall of mirrors."***

The point is, to answer your question; it is going to take a skillful treater in a joint trusting partnership, with you, to process the fragmented feelings that you have.

Questions About Diagnosing Borderline Personality Disorder

by Kathi Stringer

Question.

I have been diagnosed with BPD for years, but never had a moment of manic behavior. I have only recently been re-diagnosed with an anxiety disorder and PTSD from a trauma that happened when I was three (there was an auto accident in which my maternal grandparents were killed and I was the sole survivor, but very injured with concussion, broken bones, etc...) and another at age 5 when I was repeatedly sexually molested by a teenage neighbor. I am feeling so much better on the regime that he has me on, which doesn't include mood stabilizers. I am taking Effexor XR 150mg, Alprazalom 0.5mg tid, and Seroquel 50 mg. for sleep. It has really decreased the nightmares and increased my energy. It has also helped me focus and interact more socially. I had almost gone agoraphobic before I found this psychiatrist. What do you think has changed the diagnosis? I'm just glad to be feeling half myself again. :-) It just proves my point...keep searching for the right therapist or psychiatrist.

Answer.

I would think your energy has increased due to sleeping better at night with the help of Seroquel. Not getting a good night's rest can make a person feels as if a zombie, or I say, the living undead.

As far as your diagnosis changing, that is not the exception in psychiatry but the rule. As most any psychiatrist will admit, the practicing of psychiatry is not an exact science, but rather through guessing and observation. In addition, PTSD and BPD are close cousins. Many respectable professionals stipulate that most, if not all, individuals with BPD really have PTSD. If you think about it, PTSD is the 'power-up' model and BPD is the 'power-down' model. The symptoms have many common dominators. Yet, a vet in a hospital with PTSD is a hero, while a person with BPD is a pain-in-the-ass. It's another way to discriminate against the patient when the professional fails in treatment.

Looking at another example, consider the individual (guy in this case) looking for therapy because he is struggling with some issue that is interfering with their marriage. His wife demands he gets help because she is tired of him looking at nude girls on the Internet. He calls several treaters and profiles them according to their answers. He could approach the his selection of a treater in two different ways. (1) he is looking for support for his problem so he can tell his wife that she has the problem and she needs to work on accepting him as he is, or (2) he is looking for support to change his behavior and please his wife. Either way, shopping for a treater is like shopping for most anything. You get many times what you are profiling for. The point is, the symptoms did not change, only how the treater interpreters the symptoms or diagnosis.

For further reference, review this article for similarities between PTSD and BPD

http://www.toddlertime.com/borderline/counterwill.htm

Being 'Flat' with BPD Clients

Written by Kathi Stringer

Question
What about therapists who are emotionally "flat" with you? Is this helpful or not helpful? I had one person tell me to be "flat" to prevent being pulled in emotionally by someone with borderline personality disorder.

Signed: Inpatient Intern Nurse

Answer
Who comes up with this stuff? Being `flat' conveys a lack of nurse-to-patient relationship, lack of a therapeutic alliance, lack of positive regard, lack of validation, lack of being empathically engaged. Beliefs like that will help keep the revolving door spinning around. To hear such things must be unnerving for you (must be crazy-making for you). I would think for a person to mirror me with a `flat' effect (in a locked setting) would cause anxiousness which would tend to escalate stress levels that may lead to disorganized thinking that may finally culminate into impulsive acts. Backfired again.

Additionally, to generalize `be flat with someone with borderline personality disorder' is like saying `someone who is black' or `some Jew' and etc. Not all Jews, Blacks, Whites and etc are the same. How one person in my race behaves does not speak for me. Of course some may argue that we are talking about a `behavior group' and not race, which won't fly because with borderline personality disorder there are 156 possible combinations. For a staff to suggest be `flat' with all borderlines is like saying the countertransference remnants lingering from the last borderline personality disorder population is transferred to the new patient with borderline personality disorder. How unfair because staff is not skillfully trained. When I hear statements like that, it gets translated in my head to - "because I'm not qualified to handle it differently." Not only that, but with borderline personality disorder, staff is getting a `mixed bag' since most times Axis II traits are often a cluster of other PD's.
I have thought for a long time that it would help if a facilitator were hired for the sole purpose of in-service training to help bring in new fresh ideas, stimulate staff, create and inspire challenges within the team. I mean all successful ballplayers have coaches to keep them motivated, why not the same with an effective treatment team? I would conjecture that the extra cost would decrease the repeated hospitalizations. But of course, if I was in

the business of getting sick people in my hospital, I guess I might play coy (refuse a facilitator) to keep getting repeat business and job security.

Counterwill and Borderline Personality Disorder

Written by Kathi Stringer

Dear xxx,

I almost missed your post if it wasn't for nnn's answer. I'm glad that I caught it. It raises some emotions in me as I can relate to what you have gone through. I have read how much your mom has deprived you of a childhood. I have read how she did not provide a good reflection and especially the before the separation-individualization stage when an individual 'hatches' to the beginnings of self from the symbiosis of mother. I can painfully relate to your letter. I suppose it still must be painful for you to work as hard as you do trying to resolve this through your work on the lists.

I resolve my pain is a similar way. I read and researched, anything to understand that maybe a new and better experience awaits. That is the force that drives me.

Like you, I heard the term *borderline* in 1996, but unlike you, when inpatient it was aimed at me because I was so empty I wanted to die. Since that day, I have struggled to understand the dynamics behind it.

You were talking about a counterwill. In all the clinical books I have read, I have never come across that term. When I first saw it in your letter, I was thinking about the antisocial personality that is described so well in a book titled "In the Criminal Mind." Pretty much born the bad seed and takes hard work to reverse the belief of entitlement.

Then as I read on about the control issues, it became apparent I could really relate to that one. I would like to offer another spin on counterwill and control.

I won't bore anyone with too many details, but would like to mention a few things about my Dad and circumstances that blew any chance I had for a nurturing childhood that you yourself have longed for.

My Dad was a POW for 30 months and weighed only 78 pounds when the war was over. Mentally unstable, he married my mom, and because of severe abuse, my mom ran away without us when I was only 5. I was the oldest of 4 and took good care of my siblings. There were more beatings, more trauma, more crazy stuff. As a small child at night, I would pretend to be small in my mind to get cuddles and nurturing I missed as a child from my pretend healthy mom. 14 schools, 6 foster homes and 32 different places of living before age 15.

I bet you can relate xxx. This is one such event I witnessed at 7-years-old.

> Duepy, that poor kid. A terrified 2-year-old. We looked on in desperation as dad swung the rubber hose against his tender baby flesh. It was almost impossible to see the color of Duepy's skin through his swollen green, blue and black body.
>
> Again came the hose splitting the baby's flesh. We begged him to stop. Dad's face was red as it usually gets when he becomes worked up and out of control. He warned Duepy that he had better learn and stop forgetting how to put his pants on and now Duepy's biggest lesson was yet to come. We were instructed to build a bond-fire outside and heat water to a boil. "For what?" I asked. Then came the unthinkable answer. Dad planned to pour the scathing water over Duepy as punishment to motivate him to remember to pull up his pants. When the fire was built, I sneaked Duepy into the bathroom and helped him get his pants on. Duepy was shaking. He was so scared. His little eyes pleading for some intervention. Someone to protect him, to hold him, to love him. I tied the best I could calm him so he could show Dad what a 'big boy' he was without tears. I knew the tears would just make Dad angrier.
>
> Duepy, a brave, beaten little baby pulled it together and showed Dad what a 'big-boy' he was by drying his tears and pointed to his pants – all pulled up. He must have been in so much pain with his swollen skin rubbing against those heavy jeans. For now, Duepy had a reprieve.

As many beatings I have received from my Dad, I don't think none compared to how he beat Duepy day after day with whatever he laid his hands on. I don't remember seeing a smile on his face, only a look of fright and confusion. Thinking back, I do not remember Duepy's skin being free from welts or the shades of green and gray.

At times I wonder what ever happened to Duepy, if he survived his developmental years. I wonder what effect the senseless beatings had on his impressionable mind. I wonder if he was able to secure any healthy attachments of trust. I wonder about Duepy, the baby that never was, only a 'big-boy'. I wonder....

Back to the counterwill and control. I have the same problem. I won't chalk it up as a flea that jumped from my Dad. Although I could easily claim that, since when it comes to splitting someone bad, I think my Dad has got to be the heavy weight champion at it. Either he can't praise the person enough, or they are to be stocked and destroyed. I've seen him point guns and fire at people. I have seen him point a gun at the person I love most in the whole world, for to destroy her would destroy me. I've seen him go bananas. Seems like my whole life was filled with nutso stuff.

What did all this leave me? Or should I say, what did it not leave me. I am empty, and no sense of self. I have no memories of reflection from mother, of being held and loved. It is that part that is empty.

Counterwill can come from shame. Shame to be seen as anything weak. This is how weakness affected Rachel Reiland in her book, "I'm not suppose to be here."

> " —Don't you dare call me weak, Padgett! You wanna fight right now, you asshole? You wanna see who would win? I'd kick you in the balls and have your guts ripped right out of your throat before you could even grab your goddamned dick in pain— "

Weakness can give rise to counterwill. To be controlled means to be hurt. Sometimes it is one of the main resistances a treater faces to address the content behind the bpd defense. Counterwill for an abused individual with Borderline Personality Disorder that has chronic emptiness is viewed as protection. This is where the catch-22 comes in. I want help, but I cannot release control, to be exposed to get that help. I could be rejected, cast out and abandoned. To open up and become dependent is viewed as a possible setup for judgment. And not to open up keeps any chance of getting treatment and healing away.

The other thing I can safety say about counterwill, is that as one treater associated with Gabbard et al (APA) said, *"I know when I am dealing with an abused child when I feel like abusing her myself."* That is a pretty profound statement. A child in treatment has counterwill and will seek to 'change places' to be in control. The abused child is now the parent and abusing the treater as if the treater was the child. Counterwill in this case was a defense formed from child abuse. And many victims of child abuse are individuals with BPD such as myself.

Some parents say the child was not abused. However, in the June 2002 edition of the Psychiatric Annals in an article titled, "***The Relationship Between Psychological Trauma and Borderline Personality Disorder***" quotes extremely high abuse rates of up to 92%! And states, "Herman and Van der Kolk have interpreted these findings to suggest Borderline Personality Disorder is a 'complex' form of post-traumatic stress disorder (PTSD)". I guess then, 92% of the time when we talk about individuals with BPD, we are talking about abused kids. It makes perfects sense why an abused person would want to be in a position of control.

So of course the person that has a need to control is immature. They haven't had a normal childhood (me) to get through the developmental states. Some stages are fixated and stunted. So I'm immature in that way.

Lucky me, I can't give up control to feel love. I can't give up control to be totally open with my treater. A chance to be judged rejected and cast out.

xxx, when I first got on this list, to maybe help out for insight, it threw me at first and I was taking a lot of it very personal. And it really was hurting me. Whenever I saw generalized terms of Borderline Personality Disorder, I cried inside. Finally it became too much and I left the list. I felt angry toward Randi for even letting such things go on in such generalized terms. I think Randi knew something was up cus she left a message on my answering machine. When I called her back, my voice cracked. I couldn't hold it together. Damm. I was crying, and felt weak and ashamed for breaking down this way. Know what though? Randi didn't cast me out, or reject me….she didn't hang up. She was 'there' for me and she 'listened'. (cry thinking about this) Randi provided a new healing experience for me. I gave up control & counterwill and cried. Me, the Terminator, crying. God bless her, she is a wonderful person.

I am offering that perhaps counterwill in many cases with bpd comes from being a survivor.

xxx, thanks for sharing your views, and your history, you are certainly a survivor too. It helps me understand the dynamics a little better coming from the hurt child inside you. I can relate. It is awful to be a Prisoner of Childhood. Only thing we can do is grieve.

The Non Dilemma

Written by Kathi Stringer

There are some lists/forums on the Internet that appear supportive for those folks that love borderlines, which may really be a wolf in sheep's clothing. The Trojan Horse that can be seen as medicine when in fact could be a deadly virus taken by the willing victim.
It is my hope that through this writing, those that love borderlines (nons) can have some sort of warning that sharp curves may be ahead on some roads that masques as recovery and healing. It is a road that may lead to blindness, bigotry, narrow-mindedness and hatred.

The Non Hat

You won't find the term 'non' in the DSM-IV, a psychiatrics reference book. It is non-existent. But since it has become a popular method in some circles of identifying a person who as been affected by another person with borderline personality disorder i.e. spouse, children, friends, relatives, co-workers and even a person with borderline personality, I will make use of the same term 'non' for this paper. I will also make use of the term borderline for those individuals that have borderline personality disorder.

Us Vs Them

The formation of the word 'non' has in itself setup a framework for 'us verses them. Using the application of the word non, splitting is unnoticeably engaged providing an unyielding temptation to split a non as all-good and the borderline as all-bad. It appears to be a useful dynamic for those who hate. To appreciate the point, take out the word 'borderline' (bpd) and insert the word "Jew, or Christian, or Fat Person," or whatever may trigger you. As another exercise, at times replace the word borderline (bpd) with 'traumatize child' and then the bigotry becomes exposed. Lets work together and stop all the hate.

Fear

It seems in order for a person to become seriously involved with the borderline, they perhaps have some of their own co-dependent issues to resolve. For example, some borderlines that are needy appear to a non as needing to be rescued. The non with poor boundaries whose life script is to rescue is ripe a for dysfunctional engagement. Some are attracted to each other like a magnets, each hoping to get their needs resolved. Since they are both looking to each other for completeness, and each terrified of rejection, it makes it hard to have a healthy relationship built on the foundation fear.

Responsibility

Much in the same way some borderlines need their diagnosis to lead them an identity, some nons do the same thing. A non may take on a name like, "EternalNon". Which is sad since it is a metaphorical wall that will keep a non from resolving their own issues which they are 100% responsible and are at risk to become fixated in their own progress.

Anger and the Empty Self

Some nons have become so angry they have lost sight of their true-self. The argument is that a non must go through the anger phase before healing can take place. I completely agree with this. However with some of the non's this anger doesn't get resolved, and it becomes a part of their identity, because without this anger some nons would be introduced to the abyss of the empty self and that would the unthinkable.

Black & White Thinking (splitting)

Black & white thinking is something that children and borderlines do quite often. Once some nons are actively engaged and enmeshed with the borderline personality, they too may begin to take on the primitive defensive mechanism of black and white thinking (splitting). At this stage a non becomes what may be referred to as a post-non. I have seen many examples of post-non thinking using absolute sweeping statements such as, "All borderlines are evil" and "Everyone in a relationship with a borderline is wasting their time" and "Borderlines never get better." Notice the operative words "All, Everyone and Never." These are absolute terms that are framed in 'either/or' type statements. I have even read one post-non message declaring all nons as "wonderful, sensitive, altruistic, companionate human beings" while this same person viewed "all borderlines as self-seeking, mean-spirited, and users." This post-non painted a non as all-good and the borderline as a villain to be cast out. She was not able to see any shades of gray. It is interesting when reading a message from a post-non that they easily give themselves away in these sweeping statements. They have taken on a borderline symptom that has caused them much grief. When it is gently pointed out to them, some nons behave in the same manner as some borderlines with sarcasm, rage and vindictiveness.

Fleas

One non suggested that acquiring borderline behavior is similar to an analogy of fleas jumping from one person to another. That post-non black & white thinking stems from a flea that jumped from the borderline onto the non. While this rings true, I've noticed that when a group of some angry nons form a clan, the fleas began to breed and it becomes an epidemic. The nons are now infecting themselves along with any new members that are seeking help. As I mentioned, some of the new and long term nons wrote to me off-list since they were afraid to join in on the conversation fearing any comment that wasn't split-bad would be seen as weak. In a non's words, "I'm writing to you off-list since I'm afraid of being jumped by the other non's" It seems they are afraid of flea bites from the angry clan. I don't blame them. I don't see the sense in breeding fleas since there is no use for them.

Hurling <throwing up>

One individual that supported the non's used the analogy of hurling. Which, I liked and wanted to pursue this analogy further. He insightfully made the point that since the non had swallowed putdowns, rage, and sarcasms over time, it was hard to be logical when hurling, i.e. making black & white statements and etc. It is true that when in an abusive relationship, it can make one sick and it does need to come up and out of the body/mind.

I recalled a time (funny now, but wasn't then) when both of my little brothers were sleeping in the back of the car, one laying on the seat and the other laying on the floor. The brother on the seat got car sick and threw-up all over my brother's head on the floor. He was pretty upset to say the least. Then from smelling all the vomit, and even though he wasn't sick, he began throwing up too. The car began to stink and I almost threw-up myself and had to concentrate not too.

I got to thinking about how this analogy also applies to some of the not-so-sick nons that are becoming sicker from getting vomited on. I've noticed some influential list/forum members that are still sick and vomiting after all these years, and it's not being directed at the toilet but wherever at random. I think if I were sick, I would want someone to help me get well without being vomited on.

Reaction Formation

Reaction Formation is a defense mechanism that wards off unacceptable feelings and behavior by exhibiting the opposite of one's true wishes or impulses. For example, in some cases the Eternal-Non who is unaware of his own borderline issues wears the strange masque of the non, and frequently makes black & white statements. But over a period of time, this masque that is very, very heavy may begin to fall and he is exposed. The non behavior that appeared as co-dependent was really Reaction Formation at work. Fortunately, most non's really are intelligent, compassionate, empathic and wonderful people and after a bit of time they figure out they have become re-victimized in this sort of forum and again need to purge themselves of all the negativity and hatred.

Run With the Wolves

It is sort of an innate paradox that this behavior is to be sold as trust, toleration, patience, hope, and love. A co-dependent person (some nons) are highly at risk since they need validation from their alleged supporting peers. I've noticed how with some individuals' their spots begin to change when they run with the pack and devouring everything in their path. After a time, some of them also become wolves, tearing at the flesh of those who need help. This type of a forum is an empty abyss and only a representation of support, and underneath....the hunt is on.

Catch 22, The No Win Situation

Some nons are so outraged they have become quite adept at getting revenge with the borderline. Some nons learn all they can about boundaries and become experts at BPD, rationalization, denial, hovering, and on and on. Then with all this knowledge and experience from spinning it off the rest of the hateful clan, some of these hateful individuals encourage the more reasonable nons to put the borderline in a no-win situation. Some nons actually delight in doing this without any aim to resolve anything. It just provides some sort of eternal payback.
Dr. Vaknin [1] is an ingenious writer as well as perceptive. The following except from his brilliant work illustrates how the victim of a person with BPD can turn into a borderline themselves.

> ***By Sam Vaknin Ph.D.***
>
> *Some people here - and on my mailing lists - adopt the role of a professional victim. In doing so, they become self-centred, devoid of empathy and, abusive and exploitative. In other words, they become narcissists. The role of "professional victims" - ones whose existence and very identity is defined solely and entirely by their victimhood - is well researched in victimology. It doesn't make for a nice reading. These victim "pros" are often more cruel, vengeful, vitriolic, discompassionate and violent than their abuser. They make a career of it. They identify with this role to the exclusion of all else. It is a danger to be avoided.*

Borderline Personality Disorder

In reality and out of cyberland, there are those with the borderline illness and those that don't have it. It's that simple. There are no nons or post-nons but only those that come into contact with individuals that have BPD.

Leadership

I can understand having anger as well. I had so much anger with the system, but then I thought to hookup with a friend and figure out a way to correct the problem rather then cut their heads off. This anger was taking up a big chuck on my soul and without it would I would be left empty. I needed that anger to feel complete. Then their came a time I thought it would be much better to seek a win-win instead of revenge. This is what I would view leadership as, to bring about a win-win.

A support list needs leadership that will help redirect the vomit from splashing on someone else, or will at least help clean it up. Clearly, a lot of negativity and hate got transferred to other members.

Non vs. BPD and Validation

What lies behind the masque of most nons and borderlines is a need to be validated. The hidden force behind the need for validation is the need to be loved. Am I loveable? That is the haunting question that continues elude us.

While it makes perfect sense to be able to have a safe place to vent with others that can relate, it is sad that at times the healing process gets swallowed up in hate and becomes an identity.

Parting Thoughts

Lets work on ebbing away the hate. Lets try and use the brush that paints in shades of gray. Lets use those skillful tools to help each other instead of splitting each other apart.

Let us find the greatest love of all, to love one self so we can truly love others.

Reference:

1. When Victims Become Narcissists - Sam Vaknin Ph.D.
Author of "Malignant Self Love"

Section iii

“Clinical Therapeutic Models for Individuals with Borderline Personality Disorder “

Effective Inpatient Treatment

And the

Amelioration of the Therapeutic Alliance

For

Resistive Individuals with Borderline Personality Disorder

Written by Kathi Stringer

December 2000, Revision [B] - Pages 1 - 22
February 2001, Revision [C] - Pages 23 - 30

Letter from a helping professional

Hello Kathi, , *I've found your site enormously helpful. I work in a one to one situation with a 14 year old who has been diagnosed BPD. I am this girls' team leader and so I'm searching the net for some info about BPD so that I may best help my client.*

I appreciate that you must be snowed under with responses to your site and so I'll understand if you can't respond, however, if you have time I wonder if you could help me.

I'm looking specifically for information about a therapeutic approach to working with adolescents with BPD. I've found all the info about diagnosis and characteristics extremely interesting, now I'd like some more information about treatment. Thank you. Jen Slade

Dedication

February 1, 2001, 2:50 P.M.
Kathi, Who cares what other people think? So what if you are different. You are an individual. Just be yourself and you should be proud of being yourself, and that is what makes you an individualist.
Joanne Witkowski M.D.

Acknowledgement

To Glen Gabbard M.D., an innovative thinker and effective teacher of our time. To Sam Vaknin Ph.D. who's acute honesty and intelligence inspired and supported me. To the great writers that took the initiative to publish their thought provoking theories. To Joanne Witkowski M.D who never gave up on me and proved to me that a strong therapeutic alliance can be attained. To all the professionals, team leaders and students who wrote inquiring about treatment modalities for difficult patients. I heard your frustration from the current emphasis on symptomlogy and debatable etiology, while scarce on effective treatment. And finally, to Cristina Cabrera my best friend who held me during my worst fears.

Scope

- To review psychoanalytic observation tools to *improve staff insight* into the psychopathological process.
- To review and connect the supportive stance to *strengthen the therapeutic alliance.*
- To review Treatment modalities to build ego strength.

Forward

It is this writer's experience that no other function of inpatient care is more critical than the establishment and perseverance of a positive therapeutic alliance. Individuals on the multidisciplinary team must continually examine treatment approaches and address the patient's transference effects on the individual attitudes of staff. Some theorists may argue that derivatives of *countertransference-reaction* from staff to the patient is helpful to condition the patient to tolerate higher levels of stress and support the use of new coping strategies and adaptive defense mechanisms. While there is an element of logic to this, it should be noted that if the treater's *countertransference-reaction* is in doses consistency higher than patient can endure, severe regressive mechanisms may be activated and the result could set back treatment significantly or destroy the collective trust all together.

Perry & Bond (2000) stress the importance of a positive therapeutic alliance: "*In the early phase of therapy for personality disorders, therapists should monitor changes in the alliance carefully, addressing concerns about the alliance when it deteriorates or fails to improve.*" Of course, one cannot develop or address the alliance without the use of empathy, the ability of the treater to take on a *trial-mind-set* of the patient. Applegate & Bonovitz describe the usefulness of empathy in this way: "*A capacity to identify empathically with the feelings of others and to step back and perceive them objectively.*"

As a patient sufficiently developments trust supported by the treater's empathic connection, a *role-identification* is more acceptable to the patient. In a supportive stance, Mish (2000) elaborates: "*The patient is offered the opportunity to identify with the healthy psychological structure and function of the therapist, especially with respect to reality testing, affect modulation, impulse control, problem solving, and interpersonal interactions.*" Once the patient is actively relating to the treatment team and joined in a positive partnership, effective developmental progress will begin. It is my sincerest wish this paper will serve to enlighten and assist professionals that are perplexed with resistive patients.

Objective

Certainly one intention of this work is to provide encouragement for effective inpatient psychotherapeutic treatment from a market driven standpoint. An additional facet to achieve this cost-effective objective would suggest a review of psychotherapeutic dynamics using a supportive stance. I hope to inspire administers and professionals to consider agency waste (the dreaded inpatient revolving-door) and of course, the possible solutions. The aim of this material is to offer a straightforward explanation of concepts and functions while minimizing their complexity. Thus, I will painfully avoid breaking down theory into nested micro-subcomponents with multifaceted abstraction and archaic language to preserve clarity. Result: Useful treatment modalities.

Section One: Incentive

In today's ever changing shift in health care, behavioral health care organizations are increasingly resistive to comprehensive treatment modalities. Sabin (2000) argues that we can on longer cling to the past era of an optimistic 'no-limits' mentality. If reasonable health care is to survive, limits must be imposed to contain costs and priorities set. The Nation's managed care system we have today is *"relatively unregulated, market-driven, largely for-profit."*

A 1996 study by Milliman & Robertson in cooperation with Open Minds solicited information from six managed health care organizations. The database of the instrument applied represents 13 percent, or 16.5 million lives covered by mental health in the Nation. Of this figure 46,199 were inpatient admissions for a mean stay of 8.7 days. In addition to the short-term inpatient results above, IMD placement of the long term severely mentally ill fell into the States 'safety net' of public social services. The Federal Government refuses to accept economical responsibility claiming to encourage the least restrictive setting for the patient and prevent endless treatment. This of course places a burden on the local agencies that has spawned a heightened public awareness in a period of cost-cutting strategies and elimination of services.

As the new millennium progresses, the managerial vision or lack of it will shape and delineate mental health tomorrow. Since we are a predominantly market-driven country, one criteria is certain, treatment effectiveness must be intrinsic and ever diligent if the provider is to survive.

Therapeutic Skills

Successful companies have learned long ago that investment of superior tooling is a presquete to maintain quality standards and prevent waste. Lack of tooling, poorly designed tooling or substandard tooling leads to failures. These failures cause a loss of resources and debt when resolving or repairing products built with inadequate tooling.

Incentive to invest and strengthen the staffs *therapeutic tools* (skills) are in direct parallel to prevent failures or downtime. Think of downtime as: *patient failure manifested from staff resistance to employ tools or lack of tools, causing the patient to resist or be non-responsive*. Downtime will cause a lag or delay in a strong therapeutic alliance aimed at resistive patients.

Section Two: Lenses For Observation

Effective inpatient treatment requires the knowledge and adaptation of adequate therapeutic tools. It is an axiom that a treater must identify the behavior and affect prior to arriving at a diagnosis. Once identified, the underlying psychodynamic complex that drives the symptoms or syndrome may be examined. Observing the patient with professional tools will lead to understanding the patient and decrease a sense of helplessness from the treater. Familiar use of observation tools helps the treater identify the patient's weakness. Once identified, the treater can offer his specific ego strengths so they are available to the patient. This section will provide a review of observational applications to aid the therapeutic alliance.

Transference

Transference as identified by Freud is the patient's impulse to target the treater with primitive drives established earlier in life that was ascribed to the original individual. Widely accepted today, transference are those feelings that belonged to significant others from previously formed relationships that are 'transferred' to the treater. Transference could have negative or positive components and both are seen as useful. By way of example, the treater may have similar physical characteristics and gestures of the patient's admired schoolteacher that would distort patient's perception from experiencing the treater in his true form.

Transference is considered the principle vehicle to bring the unconscious to consciousness where it may be examined and re-worked.

Transference Management

As mentioned earlier, positive and negative transference are useful in strengthening the therapeutic alliance. For expedient results, the *use* of transference will be the focus as a management tool rather than it's interpretation as practiced in psychoanalysis. For example, the patient may relate to the treater as omnipresent, infallible and unfailing. These characterlogical traits transferred to the treater may be from the patient's fantasy of the all good provider and parental figure wished for from childhood. These distorted notions can be used to direct and vacillate treatment compliance.

Negative transference is also useful but dealt with aggressively as the issues arise. For example, a treater abruptly ended a session on the unit with the patient when interrupted by a private message from staff. The session was terminated and the patient, now feeling abandoned began rejecting medication in transference of the rejecting caregiver. Again, from the supportive stance transference is to be managed and not interpreted. (You are rejecting me by rejecting your medication as your father rejected you). Alternatively, the treater should manage the negative transference by saying, "I'm sorry I had to leave our session so abruptly yesterday. I had an emergency on another unit that was life threatening." Confronting the patient when appropriate, especially sensitive or paranoid patients will help block the deteration of the treater-patient alliance.

Objective Transference

It could be argued that some treaters present so obnoxious, curt, annoyed or burned-out that the patient responds objectively and not as a result of regressed inner disturbances. Put differently, the treaters bed-side-manner would activate the same internal mechanisms in the patient that are culturally imbued, and reality orientated with societal norms, and the patient's affect to the treater is the same as the every one else. Essentially, the treater has a lack of personal regard for most, if not all his patients.

Vignette

A 45 year-old woman with chronic depression and repeated hospitalizations, with a previous hospitalization 18 months ago, was being assessed by the weekend MD. Her impression of this MD was that he seemed curt and annoyed. He spoke quickly asking questions. His words ran together and the patient reluctantly had to ask the MD to repeat his questions. This annoyed him further. The patient felt his tone and lack of empathy prevented her from offering more information and she kept her answers short as she felt uncomfortable and hoped the assessment would end soon.

She dwelled on this interaction as it weakened the alliance. In a scheduled inpatient group meeting that evening she recounted her thoughts of this interview with the MD and made a brief comment. When asked by the vacillator how her day was she responded, I had a rough meeting with Dr. Michaels, perhaps we have a personality conflict. At the moment a

different patient said, That's a huge understatement and putting it politely. Then a third patient followed up with a response, the guy really needs to work on his bedside manner. He doesn't come off well at all.
In this vignette the MD was perhaps unaware of his attitudes toward the patients. He seemed as though a machine, like a bulldozer running over a bunch of ants. In this case, the patients experience this MD with *objective transference.* Even though it wasn't personal toward the patient, this MD was in a position to damage the genesis of the fragile therapeutic alliance.

Countertransference

Since Freud's introduction of countertransference it has taken on multiple definitions. Over nearly a century professionals have argued and assigned uniquely different properties to explain the phenomena. Freud explained his initial awareness in 1910 as "*We have become aware of the 'counter-transference,' which arises in [the physician] as a result of the patients influence on this unconscious feelings...*" Countertransference in this representation would be articulated as the treater's transference to the patient. This is referred to as the *narrow sense.*

In 1953 Countertransference takes on an additional property as outlined in Paula Heimann's classic paper. Heimann expanded the concept as a useful instrument to provide insight into the patient's unconscious. Freud however, believed countertransference would contaminate or hinder the blank or neutral reflection of the patient and would indicate that the analyst would need further psychoanalysis. In contrast, Heimann felt when appropriate countertransference should be used as the treater's internal gage or barometer to measure reactions to the patient's transference relatedness. Melanie Klein disagreed with the Heimann expansion as she felt the patient would be the target of blame for the treater's reactions. Heimann's perspective is regarded as the *broad* or *totalistic* view.

Today's contemporary treaters (Gabbard, 2000) are moving in the direction of viewing the treater's countertransference as transference from the patient colored with the treater's own subjectivity. This is a *jointly created* countertransference. This colored subjectivity is understood by Epstin & Feiner as, "*Countertransference reaction is therefore based on an emotional attitude which is due to neurotic remnants in the analyst, reactivated by the conflicts posed by the patient.*" Scharff & Scharff (1992) expresses countertransference in the purest form: "*The set of feelings and attitudes stirred up in the therapist form a model of what happens inside the people with whom the patient is in a relationship.*" For Scharffs model to work as a useful measurement, the treater must be aware of his impending unresolved conflicts. From a scientific point of view, one must consider the result when subjectivity (patient's transference) is measured *with* the subjectivity of the treater rather than a *constant* with established proprieties. This helps us acknowledge that for the treater to use this modern view of countertransference as a gage, it would be imperative to have a clear understanding of the psychodynamics that identify this dyad's complexly.

The Transference / Countertransference Relationship

Countertransference Management

As Dubin reported, "*Patients angry explosions do not usually come out of the blue; but rather, they are in response to subtle insults and unrecognized punitive reactions that develop out of the staff's frustration, anxiety, or unconscious.*"

Poor countertransference management could be viewed as countertransference activated from Freud's *narrow sense*. This is because the treater's reaction to the patient has more to do with the treater's neurotic conflicts than the patient's transference. For instance, a skilled treater should seek to establish a *psychic space* to observe 'to whom does what' during the transference-countertransference interaction. This psychic space would help provide objectivity when visited intermittently to keep countertransference reaction under control.

To serve as an illustration; A patient presented in such a way that the treater was unconsciously reminded of her brother who was troublesome, antisocial and caused a family split. This activated countertransference hate toward the patient and could have prevented the treater from seeing the patient as she truly was. In this case the treater had developed sufficient psychic space to monitor the impending reaction was able to arrest her countertransference. If the treater had poor countertransference management, the patient may have been the target for punitive measures such as withholding empathic support, safety intervention or verbal resentment. Any of these would regress the therapeutic alliance and serve to help concrete and confirm the patient's predominate regressive defenses.

Now that I have discussed the dynamics of transference and countertransference, I will construct a foundation for their interplay and significance in the therapeutic alliance. To assist in elaboration and clarification of this somewhat ambiguous concept, it would be obligatory to review the related principles and components grounded in object relations. First, before I continue, the characteristics of '*splitting*' must be examined.

Splitting

Splitting is a primitive defensive mechanism originating from infancy. The infant relates to the mother as all good, or all bad. Until the infant is able to adequately incorporate that the mother who provides is also the mother that rejects (removing the breast) into an organization of a whole continuous person, the infant will not be able to tolerate ambivalence (conflict). The infant will seek to ward off its anxieties with an 'either-or' defense. After the infant's cognation has sufficiently developed through repeated patterns of engagement with the healthy mother, the infant will began to have an appreciation of love and hate toward the same person, which leads to the beginnings of *ambivalent* toleration.

Individuals with regressed areas of psychological development are unable to tolerate ambivalence and tend to see the world in 'black or white' or 'all or nothing' terms. In object relations theory, part of the *self* is made up of components or pieces of psychic structures and these 'pieces' are referred to as *objects*. A patient who sees the world in black and white terms also has an internalized good object, bad object, good self and bad self. These 'all good' or 'all bad' objects are separated and unintegrated. For instance, the good object may be internalized as able to do altruistic deeds, while the hated self-object is to be disavowed (projecting anger) or destroyed (suicide). The following vignettes are few distinctive modes of unconscious thinking when the defense mechanism splitting is employed:

- Vignette

  A celebrated distinguished artist read a published commentary from a peer that was highly critical of his recent painting. The artist became discouraged and slumped into a acute depression that was florid with polarized thinking. *"I am a complete failure and hated among my all peers. Everything I attempt is never worthwhile. No one cares if I live or die."*

  Notice above the polarization of: complete, all, everything, never, no one, and the 'either-or' of live or die, and hated or [loved].

- Vignette

  A resident asked a hospitalized priest charged with sexual misconduct why he would have sex with a child. The priest responded that would be impossible because he took a sacred vow and was a celebrate priest. When the resident confronted the priest with recent positive results of a sexually transmitted disease, the priest exclaimed, *"What do you expect? I'm only human."*

  In this example, the priest had unintegrated objects of the good priest vs. the pedophile. Both objects were 'split' and regarded with a bland lack of concern or denial. The internalized good priest preserves and resists contamination from the bad object (pedophile), which would cause an internal conflict (ambivalence).

Another example of splitting would be a trade fundamental for most psychiatric nurses. A patient on a psychiatric unit may divide the treatment team into all good or all bad camps. A nurse with a relaxed style may be a better fit for the patient's internalized good object than a no-nonsense nurse who is experienced as hated or evil. The patient is thus unable to view the nurses in ambivalent good and bad parts and they become either angels or devils.

Section Three: Active Technique

Projective Identification

This tripartite model is where the waters can get muddy. The confusion lies in exactly what denotes the difference between the transference-countertransference dyad and the projective identification model. Some may speculate they are essentially the same except that projective identification has a third lever, intojective identification. I hope these barriers that impede understanding will dematerialize as I proceed and identify each of the components and their uniquely different functions.

Lever One:
Projective Identification

According to Scharff & Scharff, *focused transference* and *projective identification* are the same, except transference is conceptualized from an object relations standpoint. To help make sense of this and correlate the two, think of an object described as an internal piece of psychic structure from an unconscious earlier experience with a person and its accompanying affects (knee-jerk reaction). Scharff & Scharff confirms, "*Not a memory, nor a representation, it is a part of the self's being*. As the term suggests, projective identification, *projects*. As we have identified in splitting, a patient has the good & bad object and the good & bad self. To better suit our purposes for simplification I will discuss the projection of the bad object *into* the treater, albeit any object can be projected. This projection can be seen as the patient *projecting anger* for my next illustration.

Remembering our example of the patients past schoolteacher in transference to the treater, and although the teacher was admired by the patient, there was an occasion that patient's teacher gave the patient a low grade on an exam. The patient felt the grade was undeserving and harbored ill feelings toward the teacher perceiving a sense of rejection. Likewise, when a critical interpretation (you do this because...) is explained by the treater to the patient, the patient drudges up the repressed unconscious rejecting object and then projects anger into the therapist (teacher). As one treater said the to the patient,

> *"This is your anger, not mine. Do you realize you are projecting this anger onto me?"* The patient responded, *"Can you think of anything better to do with it?"*

In essence the patient seeks to disavow the disturbing object by projecting it into the treater and then thereby attempting to control the treater by controlling the project object. Put another way, the patient projected the bad object into the treater and can now identify with the treater, hence, *projective identification.*

> Example: An angry patient has an internalized object of her abusive father, then projects this object – anger, and now identifies with the anger father – giving her an element of control. As one child psychologist said, *"I know when I am with an abused child, when I feel like abusing her myself."*

Lever Two:
Projective Counteridentification.

Projective counteridentification is similar with today's contemporary *jointly created* countertransference with an added property. Projective counteridentification not only awakens remnants of the repressed unresolved conflicts in the treater but the projected object (anger) is received with an various amounts of 'pressure' or unconscious 'cohesion' (the added property) from the projective patient. Epstin & Feiner explains: *"The analyst's reaction stems, for the most part, independently of his own conflicts and corresponds in a predominant or exclusive way to the intensity and quality of the patient's projective identification."* To see this set in motion, observe the following:

> A borderline patient said to the doctor out of the blue,
> ***Client***: You don't like me, do you? I know you don't.
> ***Treater***: Why do you say I don't like you?
> **Client**: Because I know you don't! That's why! You never have liked me!
> ***Treater***: That's not so
> **Client**: "Yes it is so, you hate me! You are a liar! You HATE ME!"
> ***Treater***: "I don't appreciate being called a liar!!"
> ***Client***: The patient then said as if triumphantly, "See, I was right. Your face is red, your veins are bulging out of the side of your neck. I knew it all along!"

As demonstrated, these first two levers happened instantaneously, snap, like that. Once the treater unconsciously accepts the projected object, the patient has a sense of control deriving from identify with the projected object, anger in this case. When this dynamic is active, the treater feels as though not herself, rather as though an alien force (Gabbard) has taken her over. Her day-to-day consistent self is overwhelmed by the energized projected object amalgamated with derivatives of her repressed conflicts brought to the surface. Because the repressed conflicts are awakened in the treater, it stands to reason that some treaters will be a better fit for the projected object than another treater. This 'fit' is what is referred to as the *countertransference hook* in projective counteridentification. Note that the patient cannot project into a hollow shell.

Lever Three:
Introjective Identification

This third lever, introjective identification is what I consider the most critical step of this model. It is here that the patient's ability to relate to the world and the concept of self will be modified, a positive vehicle for effective treatment.

Recall the patient projected a highly energized object - anger. The treater provided a countertransference hook, and the projected anger now resides in the treater. Once accepted unconsciously by the treater, the object may then be *contained* and detoxified by the treater and then introjected by the patient. The patient then assimilates the modified object, which will modify the patient's constitution of self. Below is a beautiful example of this technique.

> An angry inpatient borderline female was consistently contemptuous with a resident. The problems began after this pleasant-natured resident introduced himself and the patient reacted to him with a lack of personal regard.
> Are you a resident?
> The resident reluctantly confirmed that he was.
> Oh God! How did I get stuck with a resident!? Well, you better go and read your text books so you will know how to treat me, because I have borderline personality disorder.
> Of course this interaction frazzled the young resident giving rise to difficult countertransference issues. Finally, one day he was pushed over the edge while interacting with the patient.
> Oh, bye-the-way, said the patient, I hope for your sake you don't go into your own practice when you leave here. I mean, look at the way you dress! You'll NEVER be able to attract any clients! You dress horribly!

By this time the resident was ready to pull his hair out. It was as if an alien force had taken him over. This calm young man was now seemly possessed. Taking the problem under supervision, the resident exclaimed, "You are going to have to get someone else to work with her. I don't know what else to do. I've had it with her!"

This is a paradigm of the first two levers in motion. The patient projected the object that was accepted by the treater. The patient can now identify with the treater that is now 'possessed' by the projected object. It is here the patient will attempt to control the treater who has been transformed into a sort of hologram or a representation of the patient's abusive father. The third lever is about to take place after direction from the resident's supervisor.

When the resident empathically approached again, he asked, It there anything that I can do that would be helpful to you? It seems every time I try to help you we are at odds with each other. It seems you are in pain and perhaps you could help give me some ideas how I can help you? Do you think we can try to work this out together?
[Helpful note from a resistive patient: Help me when I deserve it the least. Help me in the face of my rage. It is easy to help me when I am the well behaved, the good-natured patient, but anyone without skill can treat me well when I am this way. I need your skills, your help when I am at my worst so that I can understand and identify something better than myself. You may have to show me over and over again that I have value and that my rage will not destroy you, because I learn these things slowly and my old ways are everywhere I look, they are in my thoughts and feelings. These thoughts and feelings feel like they will destroy me so I put them in you, because I hope you are stronger then I am. So please don't be angry with me for putting these terrible feelings into you, and I hope that maybe you can do something with them because I don't know how or I need you to show me how with your actions so that I can identify with you. I try to understand your words but sometimes your words can't reach me because my emotions are asleep when you are talking but when my emotions are awake and disturb me, they are working in partnership with you, even if just a little. So thank you for accepting and holding these terrible parts of myself and then letting me take them back after you have made them softer, easier to tolerate. Thank you for helping me when I least deserve it.]

Bring to mind how the infant interrelates with the mother in repeated patterns to aid the infant in role-identification of the healthy mother. In much the same way, it would be necessary for introjective identification to be consistent to offer a sense of stability that is grounded in reality that would introduce a new and better world. The treater that takes on the attitude of viewing a specific problem as a *opportunity*, rather then a *countertransference irritation* is likely to advance treatment much quicker through the progressive steps.

Below is a concrete table of what this highly abstract concept may look like as a reference. In action it would be impossible to see this model in a liner modality. Each lever is feeding off the other, overlapped and interrelated. This table may help clarify and define this model in simplistic terms, a nearly impossible task.

- Countertransference Hook = unconscious, unresolved impulses from the treater
- Projective Identification = Focused transference in object relations terms.
- Projective Counteridentification = (Projective Identification + Hook) + Energy from Patient
- Introjective Identification = Patient self + modified assimilated object from the treater.

Building Object Constancy to Facilitate Role-Identification

Object Constancy

Object constancy is a term coined by object relations theorist Margaret Mahler and is the next developmental phase after splitting. Usually resistive patients have not crossed this developmental threshold since splitting is still prevalent and the patient is not able to tolerate ambivalence. Recall earlier that we discussed the primitive defense mechanism, splitting – the 'either-or' and 'black and white' thinking. For example, this black and white thinking may translate into the patient's mode of perception of the treater. Either the treater is on the unit or he is not. If the treater is off the unit the patient may unconsciously feel abandoned and this may give rise to the patient's disturbed pathology (impulsiveness & unregulated affect) that was temporary 'split-off' and held in abeyance when the treater was on the unit. When the treater is *constant*, returning for sessions in a structured environment, the patient begins to appreciate a sense that the treater will not abandon her. The patient over time will begin to formulate an image of the treater in the absence of the treater's physical presence. This of course is only one small aspect of helping the patient develop object constancy.

Other areas that will vacillate this developmental phase are addressing the physical and emotional characteristics of the milieu. The physical properties include the safety of the unit and time structure for therapeutic activities. Equally important, if not more so with some patients is the emotional construct. A forum should be provided in which the patient is able to vent, converse new therapeutic ideas, receive appropriate validation and as mentioned earlier, confront negative transference. These physical and emotional components along with their consistency and reliability will help develop object constancy. Once the beginnings of object constancy are laid down with a strong therapeutic alliance, the patient will be more receptive to role-identification with the treater or treatment team.

Role-Identification

The emphasis here is placed on the good enough treater rather then the perfect role model. From a supportive stance the treater can share experiences so the patient can identify and relate to the treater's success and failures, along with his good days and bad days. Through repetition the patient can see how the treater (or group) handles the vicissitudes of anger, irritations and confusion and thus give some measure as how the patient sees herself. This measure may serve as an indicator to mark areas for improvement or for validation of adequate conflict handling giving rise to the patient's self-esteem. It would not be realistic, nor therapeutic for the treater to try and present himself as perfect. More advantageous and in line with reality, the treater should present as a mature and decent human being, genuinely interested in the patient's improvement. In time the patient may identify and co-op the treater's conflict resolution skills through role-identification as a template to form her own new coping and resolution strategies.

Hold and Contain the Patient.

For this explanation, holding and containment are essentially the same. Wilfred Bion used this model for his contribution to object relations of the mother-infant dyad. He felt the good enough mother though reverie with her infant, would accept (contain) the infant's overwhelming anxieties. In essence, the mother would contain and detoxify the projected badness and give it back in a less harmful form. As a container, the mother would also accept appreciation from her infant and mirror a positive durable relationship forming the infants personality. Bion saw the process as containment by the mother. Perhaps one could think of the mother as a filter that filters out unwanted contamination while adding healthy ingredients before returning the product.

To hold and contain the patient it would be required to identify the patient's feelings that lead to maladaptive behaviors and events. Gunderson (2000) stated, "*The primary therapeutic techniques that make a relational alliance possible involve showing interest, conveying feasible expectations, showing resilience in the face of opposition, and above all, as emphasized by Adler (1985) and demonstrated by Stevenson and Meares (1992), deploying empathy and validation.*

Vignette

An 18-year-old girl recently unemployed due to her first hospitalization was hospitalized again one month later after calling a crisis line for suicidal ideation. Her childhood is marked by abandonment and rejection. Her father deserted the family at birth and her mother was a chronic drug user who intermittently put her through a string of foster homes. She reports sexual abuse from one foster home and has discussed early memories of her mother taking her to satanic cults. Has history of self-mutilation. Currently, she is living with three families in a 3-bedroom house and sleeps on the couch. She reports household members are in constant conflict and turmoil. Axis one depression, rule out borderline personality disorder.

During this hospitalization one of her peers acting in her support worked out an alliance with her. Her peer encouraged her to seek help if she became overwhelmed and would begin to act out with self-harm. Later, reacting to her peer's support, she revealed skin abrasions from scratching herself. With her permission, the peer notified staff requesting a forum for a more appropriate release of her disturbed feelings. Later that afternoon she entered the room that she shared with her peer. Her mood was depressed with flat affect. When the peer noticed her bandaged arm, the peer validated her efforts to seek help and encouraged her to continue to find more appropriate coping strategies to resolve her inner conflicts.

During this interaction between peers a staffer entered the room and stated the following, "*Nancy, if you are going to have to be on a one-to-one, then you are not going to just lay there in bed. I've got things to do and I've got to be on the unit. I'm not just going to sit here and watch you. You are going to have to get up and come with me. I'm not just going to sit here on my butt…*" Nancy quietly kept to herself and followed the staffer.

Even though the patient was able to interact and receive positive peer support, staff had confirmed her internalized belief of the rejected self. Based on the patient's childhood, her internal objects consisted of abandonment; rejection and a sense of getting in the way by being passed off though foster homes. In this instance staff had the opportunity to modify the patient's internal objects with a new model. But because the staff had impulsed into countertransference reaction, she failed the patient. In this case, a new positive modified object was not available to the patient, but instead, the staff's tone, attitude and needs concreted the patient's maladaptive beliefs of the rejecting caregiver.

Mish (2000) states the concepts of holding and containing beautifully, "*The concepts of holding and containing refer to a therapist's attempts to be a good parent by providing empathy, understanding, and verbal soothing; modulating affect; restricting self-defeating impulsivity or acting out; and generally setting limits appropriate limits.*" Had the staffer in the vignette above presented her needs in a different format, both objectives could have been met. "*Nancy* (the patient*), I understand you have some troubling thoughts right now* [validation]. *Because you are having trouble staying in control, I need to watch you* [intervention]. *Your safety is important to us* [empathic, non-rejecting modified object]. *Because we are a little short on staff, I need you to come with me so you can be safe* [structure]."

The second response to this example would have modified the patient's beliefs, provided therapeutic intervention, strengthened the therapeutic alliance, served as an extended 'observing ego' and met the required impending duties of the staff. The end result: effective treatment.

This next vignette is a paradigm for ineffective treatment when steaming from staff's attitude rather then the use of effective therapeutic tools.

Vignette

A 45 year-old woman with chronic depression was admitted after an automobile accident. Her previous hospitalization was 18 months ago for suicidal ideation. This was her third night on the unit with no prior problems other then her impression of the MD assessment. While in her room after lights-out, she isolated herself in the corner and cried as she reflected on the MD assessment and flashbacks from prior treatment in a county hospital 2 years ago. At this point the staff entered the room and asked,

"Ann, where are you?"

When staff noticed the patient crying in the corner, staff responded with irritation, "Ann, I don't have time for this. Don't be acting out at the end of my shift."

"Acting out at the end of your shift? This is about your needs not mine. Why are you here? Get away from me and leave me alone."

"Ann, I didn't say that."

"Yes you did say that, I just now heard you said that and you meant it. I heard it in your voice. Go, leave me alone, please."

"Okay Ann, I did say it, but I didn't mean it."

"You say that now, but I know you meant every word of it. I saw how you treated Nancy today when she was so sad. You don't care, why are you here? It's just about you and your needs. Just go away."

At this time staff had brought her initial irritation under control. She looked calm as she looked into the patient's eyes. However, the patient was suspicious from her verbal attack when entering the room and her earlier treatment of her roommate, Nancy. The patient was resistant and in this instance, staff had failed the patient due to lack of observation and use of the available therapeutic tools. This interaction caused a lag or a stall in the development of the alliance and unfortunately these types of incidents are not isolated. In a progressive market-driven economy such failures are costly and the survival of this agency may eventually have to yield to a competitive agency that is more effective and competent.

Section Four: Building Ego Strength

Understanding the Ego

What are the Id, Ego and Superego?

Freud theorized that the mind works from a system governed by an executive agency, the *ego*. The other two agencies are the *id* (infant) and the *superego* (parent). Some researchers claim that 50% of the personality's temperament forms from the biological givens. For our purposes 50% of the ego is predefined from a person's hereditary genetic lines while the environment forms the remaining 50%. Our discussion will revolve around the environments that influence the ego system.

The Id

The id's sole function is to immediately discharge excitation of anxiety or tension from any source of internal or external stimulation. Freud hypnotized that the id is similar to a biological organism that activates a reflex apparatus to discharge excitation to a quiescent state. Think of frustrations, discomforts and impulsiveness as originating from the id. The id remains infantile in character throughout life with traits that are demanding, irrational, asocial, selfish and pleasure-loving. The id is helpless to rid itself of it's excitations. Out of the id comes the *primary process* of psych energy and instincts that are closer to the body process then to the external world. The id lacks organization compared to the ego and superego, and does not change with time. More interesting, the id cannot be modified be experience since it has no contact with the external world. The id therefore develops and co-ops the ego to perform its functions. In order to communicate with the ego, the id must develop a communication link. The id does this through memory traces of *perception* and *memory images*. Perception of an object is marked when first experienced through the senses and then a memory image takes form perception. For example, when the infant cried and the mother produced her breast, a memory trace of the objective object was formed as a memory image. This brings us to what is called the *primary process*. Later, when the infant was hungry (tension), a memory image of the objective object, the breast, was recalled from a memory trace to reduce tension (*wish-fulfillment*). In other words, the primary process, a function of the id, brings to mind its needs through memory traces. The id is governed by the *Pleasure Principle*.

> ***Pleasure Principle*** = Aim to rid and reduce tension to a low level. Tension may be experienced as pain or discomfort. Relief is experienced as pleasure of satisfaction. In succinct, the id avoids pain and seeks pleasure.
>
> ***Wish-fulfillment*** = The id seeks to discharge its tension by the formation of an image of the tension reducing object though fantasy or dreams. An example here would be a man stranded in the desert with great thirst and then imagines a water hole that is in reality only dust.
>
> This brings us to two issues for any id process. To discharge tension thought Wish-fulfillment or succumb to the influence of the ego which bounds the energy of the id temperately until an appropriate release can be discovered.

The Ego

The ego is the decision maker, making transactions between the self and cultural reality, controlling and governing the id and the superego while maintaining socially accepted behavior with the external world.

The function of the ego operates through thinking and reasoning which leads to the *secondary process*. The id generates a memory image of an object, the primary process and then the ego *thinks* of a plan to retrieve the object, the *secondary process*. To satisfy the id the ego must negotiate between the psychosocial demands of reality and the demands of the id, and then comprise. It is this compromise which society judges weather or not a person is normally adjusted. For example, the id that demands the immediate release of urine must subject itself to the regulation of the ego which delays the release until the person has arrived at a socially accepted area to discharge the substance. Transactions between the self and reality are controlled by the ego, the executive branch of the personality that controls and governs the id and the superego while maintaining a compromise with the external world. Disharmony and maladjustment results when the ego relinquishes too much power to the id, superego or to the external world. The ego is governed by the *Reality Principle*.

Reality Principle = Aim to postpone to discharge of energy until actual object that will satisfy the need has been discovered or produced. In other words, the ego tolerates tension until discharged by appropriate form of behavior. The Reality Principle *only suspends* the Pleasure Principle in the interest of reality. When the id is governed by the Reality Principle, a by law of the ego, the id's energy is said to be bound until eventual discharge, while holding the id's Pleasure Principle in abeyance.

To recap, the Secondary Process of the Ego is governed by the Reality Principle. The Primary Process belongs to the id that pictures a need for an object through memory traces. Then the Secondary Process of the Ego sets about getting the object or brings it into existence through cognition and rules of the Reality Principle. The ego is basically an executive agency of the system dedicated to thinking and problem solving. The infant ego will continue to grow though the Reality Principle by reality testing, meaning setting a plan into action and judging what works and what does not work. The psychological growth stimulated from reality testing improves perception, thinking, memory and action. As the psychological function of the ego develops it can appreciate a perceptual system that perceives the external world with greater precision and accuracy. This growth will vacillate more effective plans when scanning the environment though experienced filters to enable quicker solutions.

Superego

The superego is the ideal agency of the mind. It is the moral or judicial branch of the personality, the inner critic. It seeks unrealistic perfection rather then pleasure or reality. The superego develops its moral code out the ego though assimilation of discipline from parents, schoolteachers, religious agents and authority figures. Consequences from discipline give rise to the formation and incorporation for what is bad, good, moral, immoral, sinful and virtuous. Through repeated assimilations from authority, the superego forms a subjective impression that develops the inner critic to keep the personality inline with the wishes of authority figures. Its main rule of function is to secure their pleasure and avoid their displeasure. I should mention here that the superego is divided up into two sub-systems;

1. The ego-ideal is formed out of rewards based on what the child perceives from parents to be morally good. Good = Rewards. Some examples of physical rewards would be toys and food. Psychological rewards would be cuddling, love, affection, and approved expressions.
2. The conscience is formed out of punishments and discipline on what the child perceives from the parents to be morally bad. Bad = Punishments. Some examples of physical punishments are corporal

punishments, and isolation. Psychological rewards would be scorn or disapproving facial expressions.

The ego-ideal and the conscience are at opposite poles of the continuum and both exert demands on the ego. The superego formed out of the child's wishes for love. Not being loved means an unloving mother who creates painful states of tension by withholding food, emotional soothing and other vital life necessities. For the superego to be effective it must exercise the same power as the parents. Like the parents and authority figures, the superego implements rules and regulations by rewards and punishments.

The Id, Ego and Superego as an Operative System

The formation of the superego reflects how a person reacts to authority figures, since it is a template of earlier experiences with parents. The superego holds the traditional values and the ideals of cultural and society handed down from primary caretakers that influenced the child. The superego serves the function to bear pressure on the ego to maintain order and moral character in accordance to societal norms. The superego is not able to comprise but demands perfection and places restraints on the table of the ego.

The id however is not concerned with perfection but to rid itself imminently of anxiety, apprehension and discomfort. In the wake of id would be lawlessness, immoral sex acts, unregulated emotions and affect, fulminate explosions of impulsiveness, lack of personal regard toward others and any impulse that would serve to rid itself of tension.

Caught between these two relentless forces of the id and superego is the ego that acts as a referee while consulting the objective world, reality. It is for this reason that the ego must be able to tolerate ambivalence and conflict from all three opposing forces. It could be said that the id aligns itself with the biological instinctual demands of the self while the superego aligns itself with moral code of societal pressure to preserve harmony in the external world. The ego seeks to be a 'good-enough' executive agent by repeating tests to make comprise for the needs of each force, the id, superego and external world. This is called reality testing. The goal of the ego system is to think more effectively, and effective thinking will arrive at the truth more quickly. Reality = Truth. It is here, in the ego, that the personality draws on ego-strength to combat stress from the opposing forces.

It should be noted that the ego forms out of the id, and the superego forms out of the ego. These three agencies make up part of the personality and are in themselves without sharp boundaries. We use these terms to describe their function in a linier fashion to help the reader understand the conceptualization and flow of this psychodynamic.

Understanding Defense Mechanisms

As the newly formed ego takes shape out of the id, it develops defense mechanisms to rid itself of conflict or anxiety. Early primitive defenses form out of instinctual reaction since abstract thinking is not available and infantile cognition functions only from concrete images. As the infant matures, he develops age appropriate defenses that are more *adaptive* and suitable for his environment. For example, a person is regressed developmentally when he predominately operates from primitive defenses that no longer serve him. His defenses are *maladaptive* if they cause interpersonal problems in relationships or cause chronic friction among peers in the work place or in social circles.

Lets take a look at our previous defense, splitting, and see how it may affect more mature relationships. Recall that splitting is a primitive defense used in the earliest stages of life to ward off the infant's anxieties. Since the infant cannot conceptualize that the person who loves him can also be disapproving, the infant reacts to his affect. If the infant is in rage, his hates mother since he does not have the cognition or developmental progress for reflective thought to resolve his internal conflict that he also loves his mother at the same time and that she is a whole continuous person. Such thought would cause unwanted ambivalence increasing his anxieties to higher levels.

Now lets examine the effect splitting would have in an intimate adult relationship. A woman using this defense would view her target on a pedestal or with utter contempt. Accompanying her distorted view of the object (her partner) are the inappropriate affects. For example, if she becomes irritated, it may progress into rage since the defended person (her) cannot reflect on the goodness of her target. The target now becomes the devil and can't do anything right, and along with this distorted view is rage, the affect. To the target, it appears she is moody with highs and lows to match her distorted views. If she were able to master the ability to view her target as both good and bad, her mood would have been more appropriate given situation. As you can see, the personality using splitting as a defense can cause havoc when engaging with others.

It might be helpful to think of defense mechanisms as coping strategies. Defenses are adaptive or maladaptive. Maladaptive defenses such as splitting, denial, projection identification and psychotic transferences are to be discouraged while encouraging adaptive defenses of humor, intellectualization, altruism and rationalization. Think of a defense as an aid to help the defended adjust to existing anxiety and tension. Certainly, treatment goals include age appropriate functioning but first the patient must be receptive in the frame of a strong therapeutic alliance.

Resistance

I find the title of this section fitting because I have received letters from frustrated treaters claiming all treatment options have been exhausted, and they are now grasping for straws though the Internet. It is simply not enough to understand that a child went though abuse since this information will not provide clues of the patient's intrapsychic roadmaps. Treaters have tried enormous empathic holding in carefully framed environments with heroic support and than it is a mystery to the treater that the patient does not improve and in some cases appears to become more abusive. The question is why? This section will center on this puzzlement.

Recall that interjects are received and assimilated by the patient in the projective identification tripartite. Now I will focus on earlier developmental interjects the patient experienced as an abused child that are termed *pathogenic interjects*. Meissner (1976, 1980) viewed these interjects as *introjective constellations* with polarized caps. One pole represents the victim's characteristics (child) and at the opposite pole, the victimizer characteristics (parent). When the child takes in the introjected dyad, the victim resides in her ego and the victimizer resides in her superego (conscience). Recall the conscience portion of the superego is formed out of punishment and belongs to the child's inner critic of a lawful, moral sociality. To an observer it appears this is a paraxial complex, meaning the bad object (abusive parent) resides in the superego, the system that strives for perfection. Since the child internalizes the bad object in a realm of perfection (superego), she cannot let go and separate, but rather remains in some type of symbiosis with the bad object. Recall during the subphases of separation-individualization, a child gains mastery of her new budding world. Through mirroring and taking back, though the positive introjects she experiences world as relatively safe, through shadowing and darting away she begins to separate, as she needs her parent less and less. The child's internalized good parent that performed from good intent allowed the child to separate into an individual.

Through repetition the child interacts with the abusive parent. The child internalizes a negative interactional dynamic that shapes her mental structures of relating. The bad object is taken in, assimilated and becomes part of the child's internal world. Even though the bad object resides in the superego, it remains elusive, never mastered as the negative dynamic is played out over and over again. This dynamic becomes a template for distorting when taking in new experiences. Stark (1994) reaffirms the patient's resistance to change, "*Intrinsic to the patient's relentless pursuit to infantile gratification is a wish to be stopped. Intrinsic to the patient's compulsive reenactments of his internal dramas is also a wish to be contained.*"

So what would take the place of the patient's bad object if it vanished from her internal world of object relations? Emptiness, a black hole. The patient's primitive defensive mechanisms are familiar and compulsive. Her internal world is reenacted in the here-and-now from her unconscious in an attempt to grant her infantile wishes for a different outcome. With compulsiveness, she keeps everything as it is and resistant to change. Through transference she co-op's treaters to play out the past with her compulsive drives, that which is known, even if it is pathological. This phenomena lies at the heart of resistant patients.

Building Ego Strength

I have thus far explained the dynamics of the ego and it's defense mechanisms. I have described their effect on the personality and the external world this matrix relates to. I titled this section *building ego strength* since I will address psychoeducational treatment in skills training, and the modification of a *closed-system* of introjects, or what I can refer to as the pathogenetics to change structure.

Structure Modification Vs Dialectical Behavioral Treatment

Modifying the patient's internal structure has several advantages, the maximum of which mitigates the genesis of the deep buried pain and introduces a new modified world for the patient. To help put this into perspective, think of a patient's source of pain deriving from earlier structures developed from experiencing sexual, verbal or physical abuse. These earlier structures shaped from abuse continue to unconsciously play-out through obsessive compulsiveness as a maladaptive defense hoping for a better ending. Since these earlier structures are a closed-system and only apparently semi-available to a trained professional, the patient's repeated defenses are doomed to failure. That is until now, but first we will review a fairly new established complex theory before exploring this concept of exciting structure modification further.

Positioned at the opposite end of the structured spectrum is Linehan's empirically successful Dialectical Behavioral Treatment for Borderline Personality Disorder (DBT). Linehan's concept is Zen spirituality combined with western psychological theory. The concept is inviting since the emphasis is to accept the patient at her current level while introducing change. This becomes a mutual commitment that seems almost a paradox, but is defined as Dialectical because when two opposites exist to create the synthesis, a process of change takes place. Yet this dialectical change takes place as micro-formations, once one change is formed at each end, reality has evolved altering the properties, and again another synthesis is required, but with each synthesis less is geometrically required in the advancement toward the final goal. In other words, we accept you as you are as long as you commit to dialectical change.

Linehan explains that DBT is useful to modulate affect and control emotional dysregulation. The DBT model provides once weekly group 'skills' meetings and once weekly individual therapy sessions. The weekly skills groups are divided up into *four* 8-week skills *training modules*, which could be taken twice each over the year-required period. The target is to replace maladaptive, ineffective behavior with trained skilled responses.

Weekly Skills Group	Weekly Therapy Session
1. Core mindfulness skills 2. Interpersonal effectiveness skills 3. Emotional regulations skills 4. Distress tolerance skills, respectfully	1. Suicidal behaviors 2. Therapy-Interfering behaviors 3. Behaviors that interfere with the quality of life 4. Behavioral skill acquisition 5. Posttraumatic stress behaviors 6. Self-respect behaviors

To Linehan's credit, she makes it absolutely clear the consequences concerning the invalidating environment toward the child. This is important because an invalidated child secures the child's emotional reaction to her interpersonal world, or lack of it. See this example:

Child: "Mom, I'm thirsty"
Mom: "No, you just had a drink of water, you are not thirsty."

Adult Version –
Patient: "I'm hurting inside and I don't know what to do"
Therapist: "I don't know why you are hurting so much, I just went over my time limit with you for 30 minutes."

The patient now reacts with emotional sensitivity and as the evening approaches her emotions become intense and she has patterns of perceiving herself as invalidated. She escalates her behavior toward suicidal ideation in frantic attempts for validation, which are now confused and uncontrolled.

As Linehan echoes throughout her work, a child that grows up in an invalidating environment will have poor reality testing skills as to what works and what does not work. (Linehan) "*The invalidating environment contributes to emotions dysregulation by failing to teach the child to label and modulate arousal, to tolerate distress, or to trust her own emotional responses as valid interpretations of events.*" Also, linked to poor reality testing is a confused identity of self, since a consistent validated mirror or feedback of self was unavailable. On moment the child is bright like her mother and the next instant, stupid, dirty and ugly like her drunken father, who in objective reality is not even a shadow of this biting description.

As you can see from this material, it generates incentive to accept and validate a patient's current position when entering the DBT program, to break the invalidating cycle, and second, to apply the skills training modules beginning with Core Mindfulness to address emotional dysregulation and modulate affect and other therapy interfering behaviors. DBT also stress cheerleading, coaching, problem solving and homework though handouts. Below is an example of Mindfulness Handout #1, one of DBT's capital declarations.

DBT illustrates three states of the mind.

1. ***The Reasonable Mind*** (This is the logical part of the mind that takes cakes care of the day-to-day tasks)
2. ***The Emotional Mind*** (This part of the mind bases it decisions on reactions rather then response, or in other words decisions from feelings of the 'heart')
3. ***The Wise Mind*** (This part of the mind is a combination of the Reasonable Mind and the Emotional Mind, able to take appropriate actions based on good insight and good judgment)

When analyzing DBT as a treatment program and its functions to create self-regulatory repertoires to tolerate stress, impulsiveness, modulate affect; regulate emotional arousal and cognitive skills management to act as an internal gage, and all of its related functions, the operator of this system must be constantly alert and aware of impending movements of measurements, comparing, looking for signals, guidelines, sign-posts and warnings. This patient must be as the operator of a lighthouse, keeping the light burning in the night least the ships crash against the hidden rocks in the harbor. Measuring, monitoring and attempting to self-validate through weekly sessions. At a glance it seems a daunting, relentless task that would consume vast amounts of emotional energy. Through cogitation and skills training, it appears to be a single source to control pain. To quote Linehan (1993), *"The distress tolerance module assumes that even though there may be a lot of pain, it can be tolerated, and life can be accepted and lived in spite of pain."* In our next section, I hope to illustrate another possibility, structure modification reducing pain without the consuming energy of cognitive measuring and monitoring.

Addressing Structure Modification – A Closed System

As we have coved earlier, projective identification and its three levers work together to modify the patient's interpersonal world. Wallersten (1989) *concluded that both supportive and interpretive interventions are often mixed together, and both can lead to structural change, that is, improvement in the basic underlying personality structure."* Yet, Gabbard (2000) found that "*..Interpretations were high-risk, high-gain..*" In other words, unless undergoing long-term psychoanalysis, interpretations by a therapist of early transferences through exploration could hinder progress. So in this case, the third lever, introjective identification is our immediate access to what would otherwise be a *closed system.*

Let's review introjective identification briefly through the writings of a different author, Martha Stark (1994) who states it this lever beautifully, "*Structural change involves the modification of existent pathological structure and is accomplished by way of working through negative transference* [or assimilation of positive introjects from the treater]. *In other words, if something good is missing inside, then the goal is to add it. Alternatively, if something bad is already there inside, then the goal is to change it.*"

This is where disappointment seems to set-in for most inpatient mental health workers. Constantly, they are exasperated, looking for change. "*I am the treatment team leader. We have tried everything, and nothing works. I have been assigned to look for other avenues…*" But the fundamental key is *not* change but modification, to ameliorate, to grow better, to improve. Often when I ask a mental health worker for the definition of therapeutic, I usually get a lengthy response. In essence, *therapeutic* simply means, "*to grow better.*" That's it. If through positive introjects, accepted and assimilated by the patient, then her *closed system* of personality structures have been *modified*, and the treater has in effect been *therapeutic.*

Vignette

This is a case of a 45-year-old female hospitalized for acute suicidal ideation and attempt by wrist slashing. She was progressively becoming detached and withdrawing due to her belief that she was untreatable from many prior hospitalizations. Supported by her caseworker and friends to be honest about her beliefs, she expressed her wish to die rather then be gamy to escape the court.

The night before her court appearance, her friends came by to wish her well with sad affect. She felt crestfallen when they departed that evening. Filled with self-loathing for putting her friends though such misery, she became tormented with semi-psychosis as she flung her fists into her head. She claimed she hated herself and the blows could not come hard or quick enough. The staff prevented her from self-harm and held her arms. Unusual, since this patient reported that usually staff immediately reacted using restraints.

The patient's one-to-one took action and called for assistance. The patient failed to respond to staff instruction or intervention. In this instance, the patient was now using the primitive defensive mechanism, projective identification. She was projecting her *bad-self.* [Her hated, self-loathed object] Staff on the other hand, had wonderful countertransference management, and in this case, the countertransference hook needed to create the 'fit' for projective counteridentification was almost non-existent. The patient was attempting to control the staff by unconsciously projecting the *bad-self*, then identifying with the *bad-self* in the staff, and then attempting to control the *bad-self*, in effect hoping to be punished by staff by some punitive measure of restraints or withholding of empathic nurturing.

Now we will examine the third lever, introjective identification.

Staff continued to restrain the patient until she seemed under control. In intervals her intrapsychic stimuli aroused and the patient began striking her face, screaming she did not deserve comfort, and should be hated for putting her friends and family through this. Staff maintained a calm affect with firm, non-punitive restraint. Brad, a staffer intermittently interjected in soft tones,

> "Ann, when you are ready, let me know, I would like to say something."
> "Not now Brad, I can't think. I need quiet, I need to focus."
> "Ann, are you ready now?"
> "Yes, Brad, I am ready now."
> "Ann, you are a beautiful child of God."

Brad repeated this phrase over and over, until Ann got it. Like the line in the movie, "Good Will Hunting" 'It wasn't your fault.' Brad knew she needed spiritual substance from earlier conversations.

Brad and staff allowed the patient that time. Staff used the third lever, introjective identification, detoxified and contained the *bad-self*, then introjected the modified *bad-self* object that the patient accepted and assimilated. In this instance the patient's closed system was modified in structural personality growth. Because her *closed system* had become *hot*, it could be reworked more effectively. Martha Stark (1994) writes, "*When the patient delivers [her] pathology into the transference by way of projection [identification], we have a recapitulation in the here and now of the negative interactional dynamic characterizing the early-on traumatic failure situation between parent [therapist] and child [patient].*"

Summery of Structure
Modification Vs Dialectical Behavioral Treatment

Dialectical Behavioral Treatment (DBT), a cognitive behavior model we have a *one-person theory of therapeutic action*, the therapist, in order to correct the patient's distortion, offers validation and directs the patient's attention cognitively, directing her to observe her internal process and the fact of her unconscious repetitions, and emotion dysregulation.

Structure Modification (introjective identification).... we have a *two-person theory of therapeutic action*, (Martha Stark) a corrective experience is thought to be what ultimately heals.

Both theories are seen as useful and have their proposes and each are positioned at opposite ends of the spectrum. To help illustrate this point I find it helpful to use the following analogy:

- A pressure cooker is currently situated under a fulminate flame.
- The steam in this cooker represents pain in the patient.
- The pressure / steam release on top of the cooker represents DBT core mindfulness and a host of other self-regulatory repertoires of gages, valves and instruments that monitor the steam in the cooker.
- The fulminate flame represents core personality structure.

Considering this analogy, one clinical psychologist at the Adventist Portland Medical Center remarked, *"If I had my choice, I would rather cut the fire then live with the pain."* Which makes perfect sense. But when entering into a burning kitchen, the operator would cut the flame and release the steam simultaneously. While grief does have its place in the healing process, certainly whenever possible the patient's pain should be mitigated through creative empathic methods and the treatment team must be sensitive to opportunities to rework, and add the missing links to what would otherwise be a *closed system* of the patient's personality structure.

Commitment to Excellence.

Considering the enormous detailed work of multidisciplinary treatment notes, doctors orders, progress notes, head counts, medication records and the treatment team's intervention strategies, staff should take great care to be aware of their impending countertransference. *Countertransference reaction* can disrupt progress leading to resistive and non-responsive patients that would risk expensive work. On this basis, professional staff working with patients should be committed to self-exanimation.

References:

Judith Teich: Characteristics of Managed Behavioral Health Care Organizations in 1996 p.1422-1427 / Psychiatric Service – Nov 2000

Edited by Gabbard (1999): Countertransference Issues in Psychiatric Treatment / Review of Psychiatry Volume 18 / APA

Edited by Gunderson & Gabbard (2000): Psychotherapy for Personality Disorders / Review of Psychiatry Volume 19 / APA

Martha Stark (1994) Working With Resistance

Joel Paris (1994) Borderline Personality Disorder / A Multidimensional Approach

Perry & Bond (2000) p, 22

Applegate & Bonovitz (1995) p, 54

Misch (Fall-2000) p, 178 / The Journal Of Psychotherapy Practice and Research

Scharff & Scharff (1992) The Primer of Object Relations Therapy p, 53

Linehan (1993) Cognitive-Behavioral Treatment of Borderline Personality Disorder

Linehan (1993) Skills Training Manual for Treating Borderline Personality Disorder

Follow up letter from a helping professional
January 12, 2002

Hello Kathi, I found your response extremely useful. As I said in my original letter, I'd found a great deal of information regarding diagnosis and the characteristics of BPD but very little regarding treatment. Following your response, I was able to put a pack together to distribute to my team and then use this as a base line when we came to care-planning our client. This helped in a number of ways.

Possibly the most significant impact or your work was that it helped my team to understand that it was our client's condition that was making her so difficult to be with at times - and not her.

As professional as my team are, they were finding themselves drawn into petty and destructive arguments, responding negatively to personal insults and generally finding our client difficult to like. This was despite the fact that she was clearly reaching out to them for help and desperately confused by her mixed emotions.

After I introduced your work to them and the BPD pack that I'd put together, the heavy atmosphere in the unit just seemed to lift. The team were able to objectify the condition and this stopped them taking my client's behavior and attitude towards them personally.

The work that had been exhausting and mentally draining before became understandable and stimulating now because we had something with a name, recognizable criteria and also strategies for dealing with it.

The impact for our client was immediate. Because the team felt more confident they responded more positively towards her. Because my client felt less rejected and more accepted, her confidence grew and she was able to develop more positive relationships with each of her team.

This young woman is sixteen next week and we're throwing a surprise party for her. Many of the staff that have worked with her across the years will be there and this is because they have a genuine affection for her.

Prior to her diagnosis we were looking at long term care in a therapeutic setting for this client. Now, because of the work we've been able to do with her, we're moving her towards independence.

Finally, I have been able to pass on the pack I put together, including your response, to other team leaders who have begun working with BPD young people. So, your work has impacted across our organization and on the lives of a number of young people.

Thanks once again for all that you do. Jen

The Rapprochement Child

Written by Kathi Stringer
April 27, 2004

This paper addresses the fixated child that resides within the adult psych of individuals with borderline personality disorder in the treatment environment. A writer's question is answered in 2 parts. Part 1, a review of relevant theory and part 2 is a response to her concerns.

- Letter
- Part 1
- Part 2

The Letter - QUESTION:

Dear Kathi, I'm hoping you might be able to help me with something. My therapist thinks I am always being manipulative with her, but I'm not. I've taken in articles to her from your web site and others that explain exactly how I feel when I say or do things, and why I say and do them. But she takes it that I am purposely and with intent trying to "get my way" by attempting to anger her, attempting to cause guilt, trying to make her feel bad - but I've never ever thought those things when I say or do something with her. I actually don't tell her a lot of things because I know she thinks I say them to manipulate her. I know it appears I am manipulative, but I don't tell her things to make HER feel a certain way to get the response I want. If I tell her I feel suicidal, it's because I truly do feel suicidal and want her help. I don't tell her that because I just want her attention. Since she thinks so strongly that I try to manipulate her all the time, I don't tell her things I should - such as, when I am feeling extremely suicidal. I know suicidal ideation is prevalent in those with Borderline Personality Disorder, (I've attempted suicide several times). Is it likely I'll commit suicide? No. But that's not what I'm thinking when I'm feeling suicidal. I don't have rational thoughts - manipulating my therapist most certainly isn't one of the top things I'm thinking when I'm in crisis - wanting and needing her help and guidance is what I'm after, not making her mad, pushing her buttons, trying to "get my way" against her wishes, trying to convince her I'm feeling something I'm not just to elicit a response, etc.

How do I get her to understand my point? How do I get her to realize that although it may appear I am being manipulative, I'm not - it's not even a thought. I'll write her and tell her how I feel and ask her to help me understand what's going on - she thinks I'm writing to elicit email from her. When I ask her a question about feelings or emotions, which is pretty simplistic to those who weren't traumatically abused, she thinks I'm asking her something I already know the answer to just to get an answer. It just infuriates me. It takes a lot for me, given I'm a perfectionist and hate feeling and appearing unintelligent, to tell her "I don't understand what this statement means," and her not respond or respond with a tone, talking to me like I'm a baby. I HONESTLY don't know - if I'm asking, it's because I DON'T KNOW, but she doesn't see it that way. I'm SO frustrated about this. It hinders me from telling her things I need and want to tell her - both good and bad. I tried to explain this to her several times, but she won't listen.

To give a perfect example: I had an appt with her and I arrived about 6 minutes before my appt time. Before I knew it, it was 5 minutes, then 10 minutes, 13 minutes, 15 minutes past my appt time - I was in a panic, my anxiety level was sky high, I had nicked my hand 6 times till it began bleeding, I was getting dizzy, having trouble breathing, and all that was going through my head was what was going to happen once I got in there. I was calm when I arrived, but after waiting about 16 minutes, the calm ocean wave was out to sea and I couldn't focus anymore. So I left after waiting about 20 minutes - I had to change my focus and direct it to something else, seeing a different view, moving, etc. When I came back, she was still busy with her current client, and since I wasn't feeling much calmer, I left again for a few minutes. This time, even though the other client still hadn't come out, I felt much calmer.

When I got into the office I told her I left because I just couldn't sit anymore, I had to refocus, I was too anxious, etc., etc. She kept making gestures and facial expressions giving the indication "yeah, right...sure that's why." She went into this big whole explanation of what she "did for me" to keep the rest of the afternoon free and to tell me several more times what she gave up to keep my appt. It was pissing me off that she sat there and repeatedly was trying to make me feel guilty. She basically told me that I left to manipulate her into ending her session with the previous client. That never, ever, EVER, crossed my mind - getting calm was my objective for what I did. When I walked in, I was shaking so bad, I nearly fell trying to sit in the chair. I was still having difficulty breathing - she finally told me it was okay and to calm down, as I was breathing way to shallow.
We slightly discussed manipulation as she was reading a manual - when she got to the manipulation part, it was just pissing me off and she knew it.

She looks up and says, "Ooooo - there's that nasty word again." I said, "that's because I'm not manipulative." She snickers and looks down at her book and then looks up with her eyes and says, "yeah....right." OMG - I wanted to lunge forward!

Anyhow, do you have any suggestions on how to get her to see things from my eyes, from my mind, from my experience, from my abuse, from my beliefs and realize that even IF it appears I'm being manipulative, I'm not???
Thanks!

Theory – Part 1

***Answer*:**

Borderline personality disorder is an emotional developmental fixation that would be age appropriate to the toddler. Before I get into the meat of your letter; lets review relevant theory to set my response into perspective.

Vestiges of theory components were annexed from a paper titled: "An Object Relations Approach to Understanding Unusual Behaviors and Disturbances - K. Stringer"

Source

This paper has applied widely accepted models grounded in object relations. The main source of this material was lifted from the observations, conclusions and scholarly work of Margaret Mahler and her dedicated collages. Mahler had secured grants that funded a major project that setup a natural framework to observe mothers interactions with their children as they moved through their developmental phases. Mahler's carefully arranged setting for observations (one-way glass) included an infant's room and a transitional hallway that led into the toddler's room. *"Thus, we had an observational situation that provided many opportunities for the observation of mother-infant separations and reunions. [4]* Mahler arranged experiments to measure the infants and toddlers frustration toleration when separated from mother at different time intervals. Data was collected based on the degree of attunement in which mother and infant were able to communicate. Mahler and her collages observed passive separations as well as deliberate separations, i.e. when mother would leave the room for an interview with staff.

Symbiosis Phase

Symbiosis in the real sense is a mutual beneficial relationship between two different organisms. Mahler's symbiosis *is a metaphor* to explain the *infant's innate perception* that he resides within the nuclear orbit with mother, and that their mutual beneficial relationship is omnipotent, from which he is the center. The infant now perceives mother as a powerful extension of self. Mahler explains the symbiotic relationship between mother and infant in this way *"The infant behaves and functions as though he and his mother were an omnipotent system – a dual unity within a common boundary [4]*. The infant's delusional concept suggests that he is much greater and grandiose then really he is. In other words, the infant cannot conceptualize mine from not mine, and I from not-I. It is as though there is a fusion that reverberates between mother and infant. For example: The infant's feels tension and cries. The cry is routed though the symbiotic system (mother-infant dyad) from which he is the center, and the tension is relieved by his 'wish' (mother is an extension of himself).

(Note: it is this nexuses dream like state, this blissful belief of tranquility that imprints a powerful symbiotic libidinal pull (SLP) in the newly formed structures within the infant's pathology. Gradually this pathology is repressed into the unconscious, but remains a force, a regressive pull to return to oneness-with-mother (a libidinal pull to be one-with-creation).

Rapprochement

This is perhaps the most critical stage of the separation individuation process. The toddler is becoming acutely aware of his separation from mother; compared to his early delusion that mother was an omnipotent extension of himself. As the symbiotic safety net diminishes, his separation anxiety gains momentum. The toddler is more concerned with mother's whereabouts and demonstrates his anxiety through *active approach behavior* (rapprochement). To make things for difficult for the toddler, he is not able avail himself as easily to his 'contact supplies' in mother as he was in the past. There is a mutual realization between mother and toddler that he can do more and more for himself. Consequently, mother's response to the toddler's anxiety and frustrations are at greater and greater intervals, and *the toddler's defense to this crisis is an active approach.* We call this rapprochement.

Separation is more pronounced due to the onset of verbal progress. Separation becomes further apparent due to nouns "mine" and "me" and especially 'no.' Of course the pervasive and intrinsic component of 'no' is '*my way and not your way*, which establishes a continual awareness 'self' that is splitting away from the symbiotic orbit of 'us', the dual unit. In other words, repetition of "no" is a way of practicing the individuality of "I am." What seems negativistic may actually be positive process toward developmental growth.

Often theorists suggest that rapprochement is specifically vulnerable in the separation individualization sequence because of possible unaligned growth spurts. For example, if the toddler's gains access (growth spurt) to his upright locomotion (individualization through new experiences) before he is developmentally ready to emotionally separate from mother (separation) then the toddler is at risk for overwhelming anxiety. Because mother is not as available to metabolize and modulate the toddler's intolerable affect (mood, feelings), he is subject to the perils of abnormal pathology. This observation suggests that is helpful and a benefit to the toddler when individualization is aligned with separation from mother. A considerable acceleration or lag in either environment can manifest as disturbances throughout the life cycle.

Shadowing and Darting Away

This dynamic operates like a push-pull behavior. In essence, the child runs away from mother and expects to be swooped up in the safety of her arms. Ambivalence is striking and evident since the child wishes for dependence on mother (shadowing) and then independence (darting away). It becomes a flirtatious game of play, of testing new capacities toward independence. It can also become an ambivalent nightmare. However, there are times the junior toddler may not wish to be swooped up and may react with rage on contact. Other times the child is permitted greater expansions that may lead to the engulfment of the void, and this emptiness may also cause rage. To the observer it appears as a no-win situation. During this period the child is in an emotional crises and cannot tolerate ambivalence.

Abandonment

When a child becomes separated from mother before he is emotionally ready, his libido reserves may not be sufficiently in place to overcome separation anxiety. This anxiety engenders insecurity and neediness.

The rapprochement toddler is peculiarly vulnerable due to his increasing autonomy along with his elevated cognation. He can no longer contain the illusion of the symbiotic orbit that he and mother operate as one. As the rapprochement toddler separates, his individualization is more apparent because reality is gaining ground. There is a growing realization that mother will not share in his quest for new discoveries at his beck-and-call. We now have a clash. The toddler has gone from a 'high' to a 'low' in a short time during the shift from one phase to the next. Some theorists speculate that resolution of the rapprochement phase sets toddler's 'base mood' for life. This model suggests that is it prudent that good-enough mother establishes attunement with her toddler to survive the rapprochement crisis.

A child that is deprived from being emotionally refueled can be haunted with pervasive emptiness and a lack of identify, or a loss of self. This is how one fixated adult put it:

> *It's hard to be a child in a grown up world. It's a feeling of being lost. It's sad sometimes because when I see other children they don't look lost. They have parents, structure and guidelines. This helped them grow and form into an adult. They went through the*

maze and arrived at the other end. It was a maze I have never had the opportunity to enter. What is structure? I remember at 6 being on the other side of town in the blackness of the night. No one cared where I was. What are parents? I can't ever remember being loved, rocked, cuddled or held. I have no memory traces of this. What are guidelines? I had none and made them up as I went along in life. I'm afraid my guidelines are not very stable since I didn't have a measuring stick that was constant in my life. Is it any wonder that I am still a lost child that is pretending to be an adult?

The Rapprochement Crisis

As the child becomes psychically and cognitively aware of his new budding world, he becomes increasingly conscious that he can no longer maintain his delusional symbiotic orbit with mother. Mahler states that *"While individuation proceeds very rapidly and the child exercises it to the limit, he also becomes more and more aware of his separateness from mother."* The crisis of the rapprochement subphase heightens as the child realizes mother is not an extension of himself, but he is rather a small, helpless diminutive individual.

In contrast to the practicing phase when the child's narcissism was at its peak and the world was his oyster sort of speak, the child is now overwhelmed with narcissist injury on a daily basis. The world that seemed as a treasure trove for new opportunities to conquer with his new ambulatory locomotion during the practicing phase is now being delineated by the harsher psychical boundaries of reality. He cannot do as he anticipated. It begins to dawn on him that he is not as grandiose or powerful as his first imagined.

The failure to reach a resolution during the developmental phase can have far reaching implications. *"As old, partially unresolved sense of self-identity and of body boundaries, or old conflicts over separation and separateness, can be reactivated (or remain peripherally or even centrally active) at any and all stages of life…"*

Symbiotic Libidinal Pull (SLP)

Matterson found that treating certain patients was difficult because there *"is still a strong internal regressive pull to maintain the old familiar rewarding object relations unit" [11].* The Symbiotic Libidinal Pull (SLP) derives from the unconscious attraction to the symbiotic orbit of the mother-infant dyad that was experienced when mother was conceptualize as an extension of the self (symbiotic phase), as a container that resolved and metabolized anxiety through her affect modulation. The strength of the SLP is a regressive force, an energy, a 'pull". SLP is conceptualized as a nexuses, a oneness with creation, a completeness. For example, this force to return, to regress is exemplified with the rival of baby into the family unit in the face of an older child.

> Here we see "*another form of attempted adaptation was identification with the rival baby. Matthew showed signs of wanting to be a baby himself; like this baby brother, of instance, he would climb into the playpen [4]*. Mother was intolerant of his regressive behavior and Matthew; the happy radiant child began to adapt aggressive conduct by throwing objects out of frustration. It was observed that Matthew had lost his spark for life in service of the mother, the influence of the false-self, "*all of which on superficial observation seemed to be in compliance with mother's wishes that he be independent and remain her happy little "big" boy [4].*

The influence of the SLP will vary depending on the progress on the separation - individualization phase. The greater the symbolic pull, the more likely the individual is developmentally conflicted with unsatisfactory object constancy. If the individual's development is static and held in abeyance because insufficient maternal reserves are absent or not fully integrated, the individual may become fixated and employ primitive defensive mechanisms (regressions, splitting and etc.) to relieve anxiety.

SLP, Anxiety and Defense Mechanisms

To simplify, anxiety derives from three sources (pressures) of conflict. To simplify, they are (1) pleasure seeking (impulsive) and the aspects needed to survive, (2) morals and perfection, formed out of punishment and rewards, and (3) the external world (reality). Depending on the source of conflict, defense mechanisms are automatically activated to prevent the individual from the harshness of reality. Defense mechanisms distort or distract an individual from the full impact of reality. If the defense mechanism(s) is successful, a compromise has been reached between the opposing forces toward a decision that enables the discharge or displacement of anxiety. However, when defensives are primitive or ridged, and the personality is rendered with inflexibility, then there is likely a disturbance in the Separation - Individualization phase that is yielding to the SLP. In other words, the inability to defuse anxiety renders the individual prey to the regressive, symbiotic libidinal pull of oneness with creation. Primitive defenses closely orbit the SLP due to its greater gravitational pull, then the more distant orbits of sophisticated defenses.

Primitive Defenses (Close orbit to the SLP)

<u>Regression:</u> Return to an earlier developmental level of functioning prompt by anxiety. For example, an individual overtaken with losses collapsed into a fetal position. An adult clutches a stuffed bunny

(transitional object) to ease anxiety. A child temporarily reverts to dependence as a relief from the new responsibilities of independence.

Splitting: Separation of internal objects that create anxiety. For example individuals that cannot tolerate ambivalence (shades of gray) will split a person as 'all-good' or 'all-bad.' It creates less anxiety to completely hate a person that is 'all bad.'

Projection: Decrease anxiety by deferring responsibility onto others. It is easier to tolerate 'You made me do it' rather then 'I did it."

Denial: Stops anxiety dead in its tracks. "How can I be upset if it didn't happen?"

Maturity vs. Fixation and Object Constancy

After separation – individualization has been sufficiently resolved; a more mature defense against the SLP has evolved. The child is able to internalize a consistent, available image and the essence of mother though repeated satisfactory (good enough) interactions with her. The child's integrated conceptualization of mother satisfies the demands of the SLP and helps regulate anxiety. We call this object constancy.

As the child matures and the SLP is adequately satisfied with the constant internalized mother object, a new dynamic begins to take shape reaching into youth and adulthood. The constant object within the youth/adult reverberates with the SLP to form a more integrated sense of self, a new dual unit. The self becomes integrated within the self, no longer seeking the maternal nurturing though the original symbolic mother - infant dyad. What has emerged is an individual that has separated from the unconscious nexuses of mother. The individual is now ready to enter into a more mature libidinous relationship with 'other', a life partner.

In the absence of the more mature (integrated) sense of self due to disturbance in the separation individualization phase, manifestations to recreate and replay a failed situation in hopes of a better outcome can become chronically and compulsively intrinsic with the individual's pathology. Treaters find this especially difficulty according to Matterson and Chathan "*They bring nothing into the treatment that will disrupt the symbiotic fantasized relationship with the therapist and thus activate depression [11]*.

Symbiotic Libidinal Pull (SLP) and Manifestations

Because SLP is a regressive force, its vicissitudes may become apparent though the manifestation of unusual behaviors. These behaviors are the result of mechanisms that were created to satisfy the unconscious demands for emotional equilibrium.

Borderline Personality Manifestation

Individuals with borderline personality disorder are fixated at an emotional developmental age of 1 1/2 to 3 years. Mahler delineated this span as the rapprochement subphase within her widely accepted model.

The hallmark traits of borderline personality disorder (BPD) are a lack of identity, pervasive emptiness, excessive anger and the inability to regulate emotion. The sources of these symptoms were caused by the dynamic, ambivalent and powerful struggle between the SLP vs. individualization during the rapprochement subphase. *"The rapprochement subphase is where the fixation becomes apparent, with the point of origin in the symbiotic phase [11].* Here we see dependence vs. independence.

Emptiness – lack of a maternal constant object

Since the subphase of object constancy has not developed within the borderline individual, he resides predominately within the rapprochement subphase. There is a constant reverberation of the push-pull behavior. A sort of "I hate you, don't leave me' or 'I run away, come rescue me' dynamic. We see this because a borderline individual has not internalized the 'all-good nurturing maternal object' (emptiness) and when his fleeting maternal supplies diminish, there is a run-away behavior to prompt the chase. We can sum it up in this way, "If you catch me, you love me, if you don't catch me, you hate me." When 'captured' the borderline individual's maternal supplies are replenished for a time. We can see this clearly when the borderline patient tries to woo and extract maternal attention from the treater. If the treater fails, like the toddler, the borderline patient will up-the-stakes, sort of speak. Note this observation in the toddler. "It is quite impressive to observe the extent to which the normal infant-toddler is intent upon extracting, and in usually able to extract, contact supplies and participation from the mother, sometimes against considerable odds; how he tries to incorporate every bit of these supplies into libidinal channels for progressive personality organization [9]. Here we see that the borderline individual is behaving as the normal toddler through rapprochement with his treater. The problem a treater faces is that active approaching (rapprochement) and the 'catch' appears as chronic, and therefore draining on the reserves of the therapeutic relationship. Sooner or later the therapeutic relationship with the borderline individual will take the normal course into a rapprochement crisis that is age appropriate with the toddler. What may appear to a treater as 'regression' is actually a resuming course of development that was fixated in childhood.

Response – Part 2

Now that theory is out of the way, lets address your letter.

Projection vs. Containment

Lets turn things inside-out for a moment to understand how the treater viewed the situation. After she gave up her lunch to squeeze in the client, she was saddled with additional anxiety when the client disappeared and then later reappeared in the waiting room. And, once the client entered her office (the holding environment), rather then containing the situation, the treater projected the ungrateful and impatient client that resided within her back on to client. In the treater's unconscious mind, through the mechanism of a countertransference reaction, the treater's impulse was to rid herself of the unappreciated object, as if to say, "These are your yucky emotions, not mine."

On the other hand, with insight to dynamics of pseudo-manipulation and an understanding of the symbiotic libidinal pull (SLP), the main and active force of rapprochement complex, she would have been better equipped to therapeutically handle the situation. In this case, rather then taking it personal, (I gave up so much for you and you don't appreciate it), it would have been more advantageous if she had provided a 'container' to 'hold' the raw and toxified objects (Bion) until they could be soften and handed back in a more attractive form. For example, when the client entered into the treater's office, the treater was holding the toxic objects of frustration, (I changed my schedule to get you in), and anxiety, (you walked out on me, what is going on?) in their raw form. However, at this point if the treater 'continued' to hold these unattractive objects (frustration, anxiety) while the client conveyed her feelings…i.e. "I feel out of control", "I feel suicidal," "I am not manipulating" etc., then the client would have had an opportunity to expressed herself. At this point, the treater can begin to detoxify the objects and make them more attractive for the client to handle. For example, the treated could say, "Yes, I understand this can appear as manipulation, but we understand that is it not (validation). Individuals with borderline personality disorder often behave as children when they are unconsciously reaching out for a parental figure (the all good object) and in many cases; this causes them more problems (validation again). We need to figure out the dynamics you have toward me as a parental figure and explore additional resources for you when you feel overwhelmed." Here, the treater had acknowledged herself as a perceived parental object (validation) and offered to look for 'more' resources, rather then abandoning the client…i.e. "This is a manipulation tactic and you are trying to control me." This sort of a response invites problems because it has the undertones of an invalidating environment (repeated from past childhood

[Miller]), meaning there is a risk of the therapeutic alliance would get put on hold until the misunderstandings are cleared up, if at all.

Ideology of INvalidation
Individuals with borderline personality disorder and need structure. What may 'appear' to be the craving of constant reassurance, is really a sincere attempt to delineate some sort of solace of consistency. When you think about it, many of the borderline symptoms are intrinsic of their shifting perception and instability. For example, splitting is a defense that changes perception with rapid and marked opposites (poor stability). Lack of identify also signifies poor interpersonal boundaries and an empty sense of self (the abyss). When we blend instability within the abyss, we see an individual that questions their emotions on a regular basis. It is not uncommon that these confused persons seek clarification on the simplest terms. As one client shared,

> "When I ask her a question about feelings or emotions, which is pretty simplistic to those who weren't traumatically abused, she thinks I'm asking her something I already know the answer to just to get an answer. It just infuriates me."

This statement is reflected in the material and work of writer Alice Miller. Her studies reflect that children who survived an abusive childhood, ended up doubting their simplest emotions. Since as children, they hadn't experienced a constant role model, they lacked the gold standard in which to compare their emotions. For example the child says, "I'm thirsty." And then came the invalidating response, "You are not thirsty, you just had a drink of water." This underscores the paradigm of an invalidating environment. The child is taught not to trust their most basic emotions by what they view as almost God-like role models.

You Echoed It, Therefore It Is.
At times treaters are perplexed when the client asks them to explain the appropriate feelings for a given array of circumstances. At other times the treater may interpret the client's request as a manipulation tactic to elicit a pathetic response (the despised and needy provoker). When in reality, what sits before the treater is an emotional child fixated in the rapprochement sub-phase of separation-individualization. The fixated individual is unsure and confused as to how to experience appropriate emotions on a consistent basis. Therefore, it is not unreasonable that the treater offer a supportive ego as a new model of object constantly for the individual with borderline personality disorder. And, this is 'not' a quick fix, I said it once, there, we are done with it, procedure. As with the rapprochement child, the renewed

process begins with constancy, repetition and proper empathy.

SLP vs. Validation, Reality, and Limits

Imagine, being an intellectual adult governed by rapprochement fixation. The symbiotic libidinal pull (SLP) is relentless; to be one again with the Nexus (the all nurturing embodiment) is ever pervasive. Yet, the force of the SLP can be counterbalanced with validation, reality and boundaries. For example, we state, "Total surrender to the SLP equates to decomposition of acute regression or psychosis. This path may lead to locked inpatient long-term custodial care at a state hospital. Any chance you have at a real life to experience joy would be put on hold. How would you feel about that?"

To counterbalance the pervasiveness of the SLP, we use intervention, i.e. validation, reality and limits. First, we began with validation, "Yes, it makes perfect sense that you need/want me to mother you, and take care of you (validation/reflects understanding). You deserve that. You deserve a 'do over.'" This improves the clients sense of being understood. Now we attach truth. "Yet, in reality, this would be impossible. I can't be a real mom and take you home and start all over again. I know that on some level that is sad to hear, but to say something else wouldn't be truthful. There is something I need to teach you, and that is how to grieve in our work together." Next, we move to empathic boundaries. "One of the reasons I became a treater is to help you. It will be important in our work together that you finally have emotional stability that you can count on. I have learned that there are some things that I need to explain in order to protect you from additional loss and abandonment. I have set up a program. I will need to work with you x days a week, and want you call when you are in a crisis. I limit the number of calls to x times a week to help encourage you to tolerate unpleasant feelings while I am with you in spirit. I hope in our work together that you can learn I am there with you, supporting you, even when you cannot see me. This framework will help provide the consistency you need and relieve your fears of abandonment.

To help you feel this structure is real and to help you feel a sense of containment, we need to have an agreement/contract between us. When I sense that you are confused and need help in making decisions for your safety, you promise to follow my instructions or crisis plan to the best of your ability. I say this because there may be times when it will not be in your best interest for me to personally handle the life-threatening situations. In those cases another qualified individual/agency will handle the emergency. In order for me to help you best, I must maintain a certain level of objectivity, and I can't do that if I'm part of the problem because I've crossed the lines. I must keep both my feet on the shore if I'm to throw you a life raft and pull you in.

Summary

It is not unusual for an individual with borderline personality disorder to seek direction and validation for their emotions. Nor is it unusual for these conflicted individuals to unconsciously experiment with the new holding environment provided for them. Stark (1994) reaffirms, "*Intrinsic to the patient's relentless pursuit to infantile gratification is a wish to be stopped. Intrinsic to the patient's compulsive reenactments of his internal dramas is also a wish to be contained.*" Since these individuals are rapprochement fixated, they will test and retest, ask and re-ask. To ameliorate the treatment prognosis, the treater will need to validate and revalidate. The treater must role model consistency (the constant object), i.e. when limits are tested; a matter-of-fact response is carried out AND carried out as empathic discipline (to learn) rather then as punishment (punitive - the execution boundary). There is reassurance and comfort in this since it provides consistency with structure. The client over time will begin to formulate an image of the empathic and validating treater in the absence of the treater's physical presence. Basically, the insightful treater begins at the client's rapprochement emotional arrest RATHER then with the intellectual false self, which is of little substance. Constancy equates to progress, and inconstancy equates to stagnation, or worse, concretes the belief that the self is without a membrane, and the client is eternally doomed to reenact their tragedy in hopes for a better outcome. In succinct, it is parliament the therapeutic holding environment is imbued with Constancy, Empathy, Validation, Reality and Limits.

References:

2003 - An Object Relations Approach to Understanding Unusual Behaviors and Disturbances – K. Stringer
http://www.toddlertime.com/general/disturbances.htm

2001 - Effective Inpatient Treatment And the Amelioration of the Therapeutic Alliance For Resistive Individuals with BPD K. Stringer
http://www.toddlertime.com/borderline/alliance.htm

Treatment Strategies with Borderline Personality Clients

Is the Treater Your Parent?

Written by Kathi Stringer

August 6, 2003

Forward:

Thank you for taking the time to read this material. Work of this sort is long past due. I often receive letters from persons with borderline personality organization that are hurting. Their hurt runs so deep that they are attaching to their treater in a prenatal way in hopes to make up for all they missed, and are still missing. As treatment continues the client's longing for the perfect parent can become desperate, in fact so desperate the client may begin to think the treater really IS their parent. The parental fantasy can become that intense. If the fantasy (fantasy transference) escalates to these proportions, treatment is practically doomed for failure if not addressed by the treater. Since a treater is not able to provide that kind (concrete) of supervision, holding and nurturing, it is important that the treater clarifies the difference between a 'abstract therapeutic relationship' (can do) and a 'concrete relationship' (cannot do) as treatment progresses.

However, there are very EFFECTIVE ways (abstract - can do) in which a treater can supervise, hold and nurture the client that can promote healing and growth, and that is the purpose this paper.

Scope

This material is aimed mostly at treating the client with abandonment and separation issues with borderline personality symptoms. First, we will look at concepts and distortions assumed by the client and some treaters (the treater is my parent) to prepare a realistic treatment modality. Next, we will move into the working "framework" and "containment" to maintain stability to deliver treatment. Finally, we will discuss a 'balance' treatment strategy to offer new and corrective experiences for the client.

Review of Identity Fragmentation

Individuals that tend to dissociate (depersonalization) are usually fragmented. There is a sense of tuning out, leaving the here-and-now, or feeling as though one is watching from a distance what is taking place

between self and other. At times there can be memory loss or flight-of-time.
Due to fragmentation of the closed core psych structures (one part of the mind is not conscious of what the other part of the mind is doing), the internal links between structures are 'split' and obscure. The defense of dissociation (a primitive defense mechanism) is an extensive from of 'splitting' to repress ambivalence (conflict – opposing forces). If both parts of the mind were 'joined' before the individual was ready, the conflict could send the individual over the edge. This is why treatment is important to create a safe place to slowly add more 'links' to diminish splitting of the mind (personality fragmentation) toward a 'co-conscious.'

Usually when levels of stress (internal or external source) elevate the individual into confusion, depersonalization can occur. For example, lets say there was not sufficient attunement between the child and parent during the critical developmental phases. Through repetition, stress mounted and the child checked out of reality and into a fantasy place that was gratifying and rewarding. Now we have a regression toward infantile fantasy, a primitive defense to ward off the unacceptable stimulus of reality. This reminds me of a line in the flick Jurassic Park when fertile eggs were discovered on an island full of female dinosaurs. As the horrified expedition team looked on, a chaos theorist solemnly reflected aloud, "Nature always finds a way." Indeed, nature had found a way to continue life even though there weren't any male dinosaurs on the island! Defense mechanisms work in much the same way. When reality is too chaotic nature finds a way for the individual to survive through defense mechanisms [1]. Treatment is usually necessary when primitive defense mechanisms become chronic and a style of relating to reality.

Silence and Aggression

Silence in treatment can come off as several things. A client may be confused and not know where to go next in the therapeutic topic, or there may be so many different places to go that the client hopes the treater can lend a hand. Or, silence can also be a passive-aggressive stance (passive-aggressive, meaning a feeling is not verbalized directly but rather with indirect aggressive actions). Silence can be a way of relating this attitude toward the treater, "Read between the lines. I am mad at you! You are not helping me! You don't have a clue as to what my needs are! You are making me feel worse because I was right all along, I can't be helped! You are just like everyone else in my life that has failed me!" The treater may try to figure out what the client is thinking and say something like "Is it helpful for me to sit with you in silence? Okay, you are not communicating, perhaps it will be helpful if I will sit here in silence with you." As in childhood, the attunement appears to have failed again in the here-and-now. By now the client's veins may be bulging in their neck and are thinking about dumping the clueless treater as rage is mounting out of frustration.

Parental Affiliation

Many borderline personality disorder clients are starving for parental nurturing and affection. They may harbor unarticulated fantasies that the treater will swoop them up out of the abyss and somehow contain them in security. Most borderline personality disorder clients are highly fragmented and the thought of containment by the treater is compulsively revisited in their mind without any ability to understand the restrictive nature of such a fantasy. Let's consider the clash of the "parental therapeutic relationship" vs. "parental relationship."

Ideal Parental Relationship (concrete)

The child lives with the primary caretaker. The primary caretaker (mother in this example) is responsible to help the child facilitate through the developmental phases to promote age appropriate functioning [1]. Mother wakes up the child in the morning, prepares food, washes clothes, nurtures, disciplines, and engages in all aspects of the child's life. And, mother does not charge the child to go through this process.

Parental Therapeutic Relationship (abstract)

The treater is paid to help the client go through the developmental process and the client is emotionally concrete in their thinking and has no clue how to relate to an abstract therapeutic relationship. For example, if a treater tries to verbalize to the client that she (the client) has value, it works about as well as disappearing ink. It sinks in for a time, but dissolves as the internal agents take over. The signature is on the contract today (I have value) but tomorrow the signature is gone (I have no value) and the contract is meaningless. The more the treater tries to convince the client they have value, the more the client is reminded later that the signature keeps disappearing. This dynamic appears to render the client more and more hopeless. Possibly, because the treater is communicating in the abstract and the client is hearing in the concrete.

Let's pause for moment a look at the source of concrete understanding within the borderline personality disorder client. In the treatment setting the client is hurting; at a loss to articulate their needs, and words of nurturing mean nearly zip. The client in treatment is essentially a child [4] when it comes to absorbing a treaters message. If the message is directed to the fake adult, the ink of the message disappears. If the message is targeted to the true borderline personality disorder functioning of the client (child), the message tends to reach its target. The fake higher functioning adult begins to disappear as treatment moves on. To some treaters it appears therapy is making the client worse, when in fact they have finally unmasked the fake adult and the developmental process can resume.

It appears to be difficult to communicate an abstract therapeutic relationship with a concrete client that understands 'messages in action' and NOT verbal messages. For example, how do you explain to a regressed concrete personality fragment the idea of abstract thinking? It can't be done because it takes abstract thinking to understand the concept. Gabbard [2] illustrates in his video lecture this problem in one of his clients, "Doctor, you are not listening to me, I only need a hug. Doctor, I know all that, but you are still not listening to me. I only need a hug!" At this point Gabbard roles his eyes during lecture as if to relate to his audience how difficult it is to relate to a client that is fantasizing about a concrete parental relationship.

Treaters should be careful that sessions don't become chronically boring, uneventful and idle with the passing of chitchat. Chitchat looks like, "you have value, you have value, you have value." The client becomes bored with this and even frustrated thinking the treater hasn't even reached first base in understanding the client.

Parental Containment

The major function of a parent is to be consistent (constant object - security) and nurture their child. There is a balance between the two; one without the other is nearly worthless. For example, to nurture a child without boundaries of security and safety comes off as homeless (abandonment). On the flip side, to provide boundaries without nurturing comes off as imprisonment (engulfment). Both nurturing and boundaries in BALANCE (attunement) are required to facilitate a child through the developmental phases. This same formula also works for the borderline personality disorder client, but modified into the abstract out of the concrete.

Workable Solutions

Prolonged Client Contact

A treater cannot physically hold a client because this will open up the abyss in the client that will consume the therapeutic relationship. For a borderline personality disorder client, it is practically impossible for prolonged holding to be therapeutic, but rather a malignant one. I view this as malignant holding because there is not enough time in the therapeutic hour to modify the vast emptiness but rather wake up the starving child that will demand more, and set unreasonable entitlement in motion.

Delusion and Fantasy

Client Delusion: – Treater is my parent

Treater Fantasy: – I am the client's perfect parent

At the onset of treatment a borderline personality disorder client usually hopes this treater will 'be the one' that will 'make things right.' The treater is usually cautious while at the same time hopes to help the client. As time moves on, the treater may give clues that are parentally attractive to the borderline personality disorder client and then between sessions the client will usually modify their internal fantasy that their treater is actually becoming their parent (fantasy transference). This becomes dangerous when the treater's 'fixing' abilities are aroused beyond the therapeutic boundaries (into malignant) to meet every hurt of the client (diminished countertransference management). For example, because the client cannot 'hear' the treaters words and only briefly take-in the treaters action provoked by the client's action, the following usually takes place.

- The treater may become inundated with phone calls (action)
- The sessions may become chronically extended (action)
- The client may try to woo the treater to physically hold the them (action)
- The client may 'run' hoping the treater with catch the client (rapprochement action [1])
- The client may "fill in the blank" (action)

Notice the above actions were grounded in the concrete because the client unconsciously believes 'action' is doing something. Action is perceived as moving somewhere but unemotional words are viewed as stagnating chitchat. As we move through the work we will see how words can be transformed into action by the skillful treater.

Engineering and Planning

I have often heard these words, "Kathi, you are able to help so many people. How is it that you cannot help yourself?" My usual response goes something like this, "There is a lot of difference between designing and building Disneyland (outside) then actually spending a day in the park enjoying the rides (inside). For example, "how can an expert brain surgeon operate on herself?" She can't. The best she can hope for is to find a qualified and experienced surgeon. What I'm speaking of here is Winnicott's vision of the 'holding environment.' And I often hear, "Why don't you just say what you need?" I return the question, "Does it feel better to get flowers unexpectedly or after you request them?" The answer has always been "to get surprised with the flowers, because that way, it really counts". A savvy treater will have insight to this strategy and will design and operate the holding environment along these lines, because a client's behavior is usually a dead give-a-way as to what they need.

Therapeutic Containment

A treater may wonder, "How do I figure out what the client needs?" If the treater understands the client has borderline personality disorder, the designing process of the holding environment can begin immediately. Even though there are 156 possible symptomatic combinations for Borderline Personality Disorder, there are common hallmarks that rise out of the mix. Ridged personality traits, underlying anger, emotional instability and problems with impulsivity (See ya! I was looking for a treater when I walked in here, and I'm looking for one now!). All of which leads to a common therapeutic theme, which is 'containment'.

Therapy Interfering Acting Out

A frustrated treater may pull out this wildcard "This is therapy interfering behavior" after an argument breaks out and the treater is unable to navigate the dilemma to a successful therapeutic advancement. The unskillful use of this wildcard can setback treatment because it can come off as "the last resort of the incompetent" which, many times is usually the case. For example, a client picked up on an attitude within the treater that the client had experienced in the past that was connected to severe emotional abuse. Accordingly, the client's emotions rise (fusion ready [1]) and the client's repressed anger that is linked to treater's attitude is resurrected from the client's past. We now have a Grade-A negative transference brewing the holding environment. A savvy treater will realize this energy (turbo advancement) is useful to act as a modifier toward healing.

Vignette

During the hospital intake a borderline personality disorder inpatient client expressed that she could not handle being put into a group with child abusers. However, because the client was 'well-read and informative' she was put into the abuser group because it was thought 'she could handle it.' During the group session things got too graphic (child molestation) and this triggered the client and she left the group feeling unheard. She was shaking (transference in the works) when she related the group discussion to the program manager. The program manager promised it wouldn't happen again. The following day the 'abused survivors' (women) were combined with 'child molestation offenders' (men) in a role-play session due to the small group size. During a role-play a child molester pretended to talk to his sexual abusive uncle that molested him as a child. He said, "Uncle, you messed me up. When you fondled me (very graphic) you MADE ME do this to others when I grew up." The borderline personality disorder client immediately left the room. Later that day the client had a private session with the inpatient treater.

Treater: "You look upset."
Client: "I am upset. Something happened in group and I am very angry about it."
Treater: "What happened?"
Client: "I felt used. I felt used in the service of this hospital."
Treater: "How so?"
Client: "I told the intake person I could not handle being put in the same group as the offenders and she felt I could handle it. I couldn't. Then, the next day I was exposed to the same graphic material. Not only that, but the person wouldn't take responsibility for his actions and blamed it on this uncle that "he made him do it!" I am so angry with that. Why did I have to hear that? Why was I exposed again after I made it clear it triggered me?" (Full activated transference)
Treater: "We feel it is good for the offender to face victims for insight."
Client: "If I stayed in the group, he wouldn't like what I would have to say."
Treater: "You should had stayed and told him how it affected you and he could have learned from your views, and you would have been able to vent."
Client: "Are you kidding me? I would have blown the guy out of the water. He Made Me? What kind of statement is that? By exposing him to my anger, I would have traumatized him to a point there would be no way out."
Treater: "Then that would be inappropriate.
Client: "Exactly, then why was I put in there with him?"
Treater: "We are not getting anywhere, we need to move on."
Invalidated Client: "I was told that what is said in group, stays in group unless we discuss it with our treaters. I have no one to talk to but you. The other staff is too busy."
Treater: "What do you want me to say?"
Hopeless Client: "I have to tell you what to say?"
Treater: "The group is over. Nothing can be done. We need to move on."
Client: "But I'm still very angry about this."
Treater: "This is therapy interfering behavior. We need to move on."
Frustrated Client: "I can't move on. I'm angry. I feel invalidated." (Near tears).

***Treater*:** "We need to move on. This is therapy interfering acting out."
Confused Client: "I can't move on!"
***Treater*:** "What do you want me to say?"
***Client*:** "You want me to ask for my own flowers?"
***Treater*:** "What?"
***Angry Client*:** "How about the ABC's of therapy? How about validating what just happened to me?"
***Treater*:** "What do you mean?"
***Angry Client*:** "How about, Ann, I'm sorry that happened to you. If it had happened to me, I would be upset too. Let's talk about why it upset you so much and see what is behind that."
***Treater*:** "But I didn't say that and if I did say it now it wouldn't matter as much to you."
***Misunderstood Client*:** "Right, because I had to ask for the flowers."
***Treater*:** "What?"

In vignette above, the treater blew it. The treater had a chance to work with the client's aroused angry feelings that were amplified and connected to old unresolved angry feelings from the past (a prime negative transference). Between the problems in group and the treater claiming the client's anger was therapy interfering (pulling the incompetent wild card), the anger concreted the client's beliefs the world is bad, and a chance at being understood is hopeless. Had the treater validated the client in the mist of the anger (height of the negative transference), most of that energy could have been modified into a healing experience.

The Container and Framework

This is the first step, the construction of the operating framework. There are parameters in which the therapeutic work can be carried out. The use of the word 'rules' seems harsh and invites challenge. For example: "This is not within the parameters of our working relationship" (reminded of agreement -problem solving) comes off better then "you are breaking the rules" (accusatory - defensive)

After intake and getting the client's history we move to the next step, which is to establish a micro therapeutic alliance [6].

For example: <u>Framework (Plan A)</u>

***Treater*:** Have you ever trusted anyone?
***Client*:** No, I trust no one. People cannot be trusted for the most part.
***Treater*:** Did you trust your last treater?

***Client*:** Not all the way. I held back in places.
***Treater*:** Okay, do you trust your best friend?
***Client*:** For the most part, almost all the way.
***Treater*:** "I can't ask for more then that. You will learn to trust me at least as much as your best friend. I realize it will take some time, and I expect you will test me, but you will learn to trust me."
***Client*:** I don't play those games. I don't and won't test.
***Treater*:** In any case, you will find out I can be trusted. Are you willing to give me that chance?
***Client*:** I want too.
***Treater*:** That's good enough for me. I'll take it.

The example above, the treater focused on trust. Even though the client was ambivalent and 'gun-shy' on the issues of trust, the treater provided the genesis of consistency, (formation of the constant object), "You will learn to trust me." This exchange was attractive to the client and enabled the treater to proceed to the next step; to establish a JOINT agreement that the client is in treatment to get help [6].

***Treater*:** I don't know you well enough to know what you need right now, because every person is different, but I will learn. Does that seem fair to you?
***Client*:** Yes
***Treater*:** (nodding) I have learned that when working with clients it is helpful to establish constancy, structure and a routine.
***Client*:** That's one of my problems. The way I feel about myself, I don't really care about even establishing structure.
***Treater*:** Are you here because you hope I can help you?
***Client*:** Kind of.
***Treater*:** Would it be fair to suggest there is a part of you that wants very much to get better even though a bigger part may not want too?
***Client*:** Sometimes I can feel that part, like right now.
***Treater*:** (nodding) That is the part I hope will keep you coming into treatment so I can work with the bigger, sadder, and more hurtful parts of you and help them feel better. Do you think you are able to do that?
***Client*:** I want too.
***Treater*:** Are you willing to give it a try?
***Client*:** I want too. (Very long pause) Yes, I want to try.
***Treater*:** (nodding) I'm glad that you decided to try. I congratulate you.

The treater has explained the framework identifiers in advance and has established the beginning of a working relationship. Next, the treater must establish a treatment time that should remain constant in day and time to help the client develop a feeling of containment (a feeling of being held). Once treatment the schedule and frequency are worked out, the treater explains what they need (empathically!) from the client, which is basically to come into treatment (no matter how bad the client feels), and aim to be on time, and make an effort on some level to work with the treater, if only a little. Half the work is just showing up!

The Framework Summary: (Plan A)

- Treater leadership – "You will learn to trust me"
- The client admits to needing help
- The treater is engaged (you will test me)
- The client agrees to come into treatment no matter how badly they feel

The Container (Plan B)

The container (Bion) 'contains' the framework of the therapeutic treatment AND contains the client. The container is a membrane that 'holds' the client. This 'holding membrane' can be much more effective than the physical holding of the client.
If a container is not 'constant' it is basically worthless and can setback treatment until the client believes the container has been repaired. Beware treater; the client will inspect (repeated testing of the repairs) the container before treatment is able to advance. In essence, a faulty container can make the treater work 10 times harder! For example, a suspicion of a faulty track containing a roller coaster car is likely to get exanimation through a magnifying glass.

It may be helpful for the treater to discuss with the client (in a nurturing way) how the container works with safety issues. For example, "If you do A, I will follow up with B, and this not a punishment (penalty), but rather a consequence to keep you safe and to help you learn" (discipline), OR, "If you unable to control yourself 'A', for safety reasons, I will have to take control by doing "B."
There is no malice involved here, but rather a demonstration of constancy that was not modeled in the past with the client (constant object). This is also a corrective experience.

Vignette

Gabbard [2] illustrates a segment of the container perfectly in his APA video lecture.

***Client*:** I can't understand it. I don't know what the big deal is.

***Treater*:** What are you talking about?

Client: I keep getting put into the hospital and it messes up my job. I think I am one of the higher function people out there. This doesn't make any sense to me.
Treater: What do you think you are doing to end up in there?
Client: I don't know. Except sometimes I cut on myself.
Treater: You don't think that is a reason for being hospitalized?
Client: No. I mean the cuts are not life threatening. It's just something that I do from time-to-time. I don't know what the big deal is.
Treater: Well, in our culture, we view people that cut themselves as needing immediate treatment in a secure environment. Hospitalization is simply the result of the consequences of self-harm in our society.

In this vignette the client had a rather bland lack of denial that cutting resulted in hospitalization. The treater however, concreted the link between cutting and hospitalization. This awareness promoted the framework of treatment AND contained the client. The treater was able to demonstrate to the client that self-dangerous behaviors are a no-brainer toward more extreme measures of containment that are carried out as-matter-fact. Therapeutic Parameters, Active engagement and Consistency (PAC Container) are key toward effective containment for growth.

The Therapeutic Tools

Goals vs. Vector

At times the word 'goals' can arouse ambivalence toward self-destruction, and invites self-sabotage in the client with borderline personality disorder. In cases like this the word 'vector' is helpful. Vector is not a goal, but a looking in direction of, a setting the feet on a path of. Vector is a journey in the right direction and not the destination. Vector helps promote positive alliance in a positive aimed direction rather then the destination-based risk to failure.

Don't Cheat

A famed treater advocated that blackmailing the client to get them to be treatment compliment might be necessary. Her strategy was to FIRST develop a STRONG therapeutic alliance and then threaten to dump the client (the execution boundary [5]) if they failed to improve. She reasoned that a client might not want improve to keep the treatment going, in which case the treater should say, "If you don't improve, you will lose me much quicker!"

This strategy certainly challenges the concept of trust! It can come off as a cheater that changes the rules as they go. This can certainly be viewed as a cowardly sneak attack. A tactic like this could possibly explain why there is a dropout rate for the more sensitive borderline personality disorder clients that have a history of being abusively manipulated by others. The strong therapeutic alliance got mirrored back to the client abusively in much the same way it was mirrored back to the child in service of the parent to keep the parent's love. A scheme like this can trigger and amplify similar anger within the client that is still not resolved from the past (mistrust transference). The treater could step on a transference destructive landmine and blow up the therapeutic alliance. Use caution.

Two techniques for Change (modification)

One technique would be to address the thought process (cognitive) and the other would be to provide a corrective experience for the client (psychodynamic). Cognitive and psychodynamic models can bring about change while 'supportive therapy' may help the client continue to function without any real change. It is important the treater has knowledge of the cognitive as well the psychodynamic methods for maximum therapeutic benefit for the client. Lets look at this metaphor for clarification:

> There is a steam kettle on a stove with a large fire under it. There are several pressure gages on the lid of the kettle that are maxed out.
>
> The fire represents the source (closed core objects) of all the emotional hurts that are walled off and deep inside the client (unconscious). The steam kettle represents the person (self) and the steam represents the PAIN inside the person. The gages on the steam kettle when adjusted allow steam (pain) to escape and release some pressure.
>
> Now, the steam kettle is ready to blow at any second. Lets look at our options to keep the steam kettle from blowing up:
>
> 1. We could adjust all the steam gages (cognitive management) or;
> 2. We could cut the fire (source of the pain) or,
> 3. We could cut the fire AND adjust the gages for maximum release of pain.

An effective treatment approach is much like the metaphor above. The cognitive approach (think it out) will help get problems under control based in the here-and-now (releasing pain), but are not as likely to cut the unconscious source of the pain that a corrective experience from the treater can provide (The skillful use of introjective identification to offer modified objects to the client for assimilation). For the corrective experience psychodynamic treatment is useful (cutting the source of the pain). Marsha Linahan has taken Arroan Beck's (the originator [3]) theories of cognitive behavior therapy (CBT) and modified it to treat the borderline personality. Her version added Zen into the package and she termed it Dialectical Behavior Treatment (DBT). She has outlined her treatment approach much like a decision-making flow chart. For example, "Is the client doing 'A' or 'B'? If 'A', do this, if 'B' do that." On the upside, the great thing about a flow chart is that it takes a lot of guesswork out of how to help the client. The down side is that it limits the skillful use of creativity to recreate an environment to address the old pain that drives the behaviors. Rule of thumb, cognitive treatment can 'manage' the pain, and psychodynamic treatment can 'eliminate' the pain. Therefore, it is usually best to manage the pain (DBT) [7] while the treater is also trying to eliminate the pain (psychodynamic).

Examine Cognitive Positions (1)

The cognitive treater's job is to educate the client about the 3-way linkage that 'thoughts drive emotions, and emotions drive behaviors.' The cognitive treater also challenges the beliefs of the client to sort out any 'distortions' that may be driving the emotions into behaviors (unraveling transferences). The cognitive treater also educates the client to 'respond' (think) rather than to 'react' (knee-jerk) to situations (use of the wise mind). When addressing possible cognitive distortions (transferences) it works out much better when the treater 'invites' the client to try on different perspectives through exploration rather than to demand the perspective compliance of the treater. There is nothing worse (figuratively speaking) when a treater goes into a battle with the client and takes a stance the client is massively distorting everything. This is an evasive way to invalidate the client all over again (creates mistrust). This creates a situation where each of the participants are at odds with each other and the situation is advancing toward a static power struggle (resentment and going nowhere). It is a MUCH wiser approach to 'guide' a client toward a possible distortion, examine it, play around with it, and try it on for size. This way, the client 'owns' it; rather fight the perception of the treater (the invalidating object).

Modify Old Beliefs Through Corrective Experience. (2)

A treater is working with a client's head (cognitive – thinking) AND is also working with their heart (complex emotions). For example, many of us have had to make tough relationship decisions based on information from our head vs. our heart. Usually the heart says to 'stay' in the relationship and the head says to 'run as fast as you can.' This creates ambivalence (opposing thoughts).

The problem with an exclusive cognitive (thinking) approach toward therapy (addressing ambivalence and distortions) is that it only addresses the head and NOT the heart. Emotions should not, and cannot be ignored. Still, a cognitive behavior treater may say, "We do address emotions. We help the client examine their thought process of how and where these emotions are stirred up. We try to trace where the emotions are coming from and if we find distortions in the client's thinking, it helps the client understand their thought process, and then they feel better. Then the client is able to relate to people in a cognitive way that establishes a better working relationship. This process snowballs in all parts of their lives until most of their problems diminish." However, many of us that have fallen in love and have been crushed on the other end would beg to differ. A broken heart hurts no matter what rational views or evidence is offered to help mind rationalized away the hurt. Hurt is hurt regardless of all any 'cognitive" explanations to mitigate the damage. The psychodynamic models addresses the old hurts that are still very much alive within the heart (closed core objects).

To address the source of the client's pain, the treater must be aware of emotions that are stirred up in the therapeutic relationship. When the client's emotions are stirred up toward the treater based on previous experiences in the past from others, we have transference in the works [3]. Transference is resurrected emotions that were previously directed toward others and is now directed toward the treater. Since no situation is EXACTLY the same, transference is ALWAYS a distortion. However, even though the current situation with the therapist is distorted, it is still extremely useful to provide a vehicle for a corrective experience. This can be an intense and emotionally involved role-play toward a better outcome. The client resurrects the pain from the past (forming a transference) and the treater is the role target (transference target). As the role-play unfolds, emotions can get worked up. Then, with perfect timing, the treater can turn some of that anger or neediness into healing (modify the internal object).

Treatment Red Flags

Remember, transference is always a distortion of the client's thoughts from the past attributed toward the treater. Countertransference is basically the old feelings aroused in the treater due to the client's transference (the narrow sense).

Several Transference and Countertransference Examples

> ***Transference***: The treater will be my perfect parent. I have hoped to find this my whole life.

***Countertransference*:** I will parent this client like a real parent because I remember how bad I felt when my mom was away for a year when I was little.
***Problem*:** A real concrete parent/child relationship is impossible because the treater's limited resources are not available. Most treaters have existing caseloads and responsibilities to their families, and to themselves.

***Transference*:** My treater will attend to my every need and to my every hurt, no matter when, just like my aunt used to do for me one summer when I was little.
***Countertransference*:** I can make any exception for my client on any day and at any time. I have the ability to 'perfect' treater. I can do anything because my parents raised me that way.
***Problem*:** If this trend begins to develop, the treater is getting setup to be victimized by the client (3 AM Phone calls every other night). According, the defeated treater may begin avoiding the client [2] and swing completely in the other direction. This can retraumatize the client because the treater is now in the neglecting role of the original abuser, and the cycle continues whereby concreting the client's beliefs "I am bad, I don't matter." This dynamic personifies the treater's narcissist countertransference since they are toying with grandiose fantasies of 'all-serving.' Of course addressing isolated or rough spots is helpful for the client and is encouraged, however, be prudent of a developing malignant pattern that can destroy the therapeutic alliance.

***Transference*:** I hate my treater because she never holds me, and she is like all the rest that never listened to me when I needed nurturing as a child.
***Countertransference*:** I need to start holding my client so I can get through to her because I can recall what that feeling feels like.
***Problem*:** Prolonged and physically holding the client can open up a can of worms because this can be an expansion of the abyss that already resides in the client. It would be like serving dinner to a starving person and after the first bite the dinner is taken away. Where is the satisfaction in that? There is not enough time in the treatment hour to address the devastation of pain with holding. Abstract 'holding' with 'containment' is much more therapeutic.

***Transference*:** I really hate you right now. You are like my abusive foster home.

***Countertransference*:** Based on the way you are acting right now, you deserved what you got. Perhaps if you had understood your abuser more, none of this would have happened. Perhaps I should advise you to apologize the abuser.

***Problem*:** This shifts the responsibility from the offender to his prey. The abused must have done something to bring about their own maltreatment - or simply were emotionally "unavailable" to help the abuser with his problems. Healing is guaranteed if only the victim were willing to participate in a treatment plan and communicate with the abuser [8].

Summery:

- A personality that dissociates is usually fragmented.
- Silence can be aggression toward the treater.
- An Ideal Parental Relationship (concrete) is unrealistic.
- A Parental Therapeutic Relationship (abstract) can modify a client's core beliefs and can be VERY therapeutic.
- A BALANCE between Framework and Containment of Treatment are key.
- Prolonged contact with the client can wake up demanding entitlement.
- The treater is not the client's actual child.
- Being 'surprised' with flowers is better then asking for them at times.
- At the onset of a diagnosis of BPD at treater can begin constructing the containment process.
- Taking a stance of "This Therapy Interfering Acting Out" to avoid a challenge can be viewed in some cases as the

incompetent 'wildcard.'

- Viewing the treatment environment as 'parameters' invites problem solving, whereas 'Rules' suggest an accusatory and defensive stance.

- Goals can wake up old experiences of failure, whereas, a Vector aims in the direction of improvement and can diminish the 'goal anxiety' of failure.

- For every plan 'A', have a plan 'B' to maintain a constant container. Be consistent!

- "Blackmail" therapy can come across as a cheater, and magnify mistrust.

- Cognitive therapy leans more toward managing pain, and psychodynamic therapy leans more toward pain elimination. Both are useful.

- Transferences and Countertransferences need to be monitored by the treater. And understandings of these dynamics are also helpful for the client.

Conclusion

Hopefully this work has stimulated the client and the treater. This material has taken the task to articulate the difference between a therapeutic relationship vs. a malignant relationship. In a therapeutic relationship emotions are aroused for change (modification) because the container is strong (every plan A has a plan B) and balanced with the operating framework (the modifer). A maligment relationship is harmful because distortions are not addressed, the container is flawed and powerful emotions are not modified into healing (negative transferences are not channeled to modify closed core objects within the client).

To The Client

Please be careful that a parental fantasy toward the treater does not turn into an unmanageable obstacle. Use this material to keep a healthy perspective. Let healing work for you based on your aroused emotions facilitated by a skillful treater.

References:

1. An Object Relations Approach to Understanding Unusual Behaviors and Disturbances - Kathi Stringer (2003)
http://www.toddlertime.com/general/disturbances.htm
2. An Object Relations Approach to Understanding Unusual Behaviors and Disturbances - Kathi Stringer (2003)
http://www.toddlertime.com/general/disturbances.htm
3. Integrated Treatment of Borderline Personality Disorder - Glen O. Gabbard, M.D.
4. Prisoners of Hate - Aaron T. Beck, M.D.
5. I Hate You, Don't Leave Me - Jerold J. Kreisman M.D.
6. Borderline Hatred and the Execution Boundary - Kathi Stringer
http://www.toddlertime.com/borderline/execution-boundary.htm
7. Technique used by Tracy Shockey MSW
8. Cognitive Behavior Treatment of Borderline Personality Disorder - Marsha Linehan Ph.D.
9. Malignant Self Love - Narcissism Revisited, Sam Vaknin, Ph.D.
http://samvak.tripod.com/archive44.html

An Object Relations Approach to Understanding Projective Identification and Borderline Personality Disorder

Written by Kathi Stringer

Forward by Sam Vaknin, Ph.D
Author of: Malignant Self Love:Narcissism Revisited

The defense mechanism known as "projective identification" is by far the most difficult to fully comprehend. It is an agglomerate of earlier and more primitive mechanisms such as "splitting". But, as opposed to all other defense mechanisms - it seeks to co-opt another person to carry out some of its functions. In this respect, it is, indeed, a NARCISSISTIC defense mechanism. The narcissist seeks to incorporate others into his psychic makeup and to co-opt them into performing ego functions for him.

Kathi Stringer did a brilliant job in elucidating the three intertwined levers of the projective defenses: projective identification (PI), counter-projective-identification (CPI) and Introjective Identification. This tripartite model makes it easy to disentangle the roles of the projecting patient and the counter-projecting therapist ("treater" in the original). It is an intricate and subtle dance of aggression ("bad object") and counter-aggression, neediness and rejection, attraction and repulsion, assignment of roles and their assumption, assimilation and denial, insight and cognitive distortions. It is a hall of mirrors.

As in any hall of mirrors, reality gets distorted and confusion is inevitable. Kathi guides us firmly but gently through this maze into the dawning realization of who does what and to whom. It is an astounding journey and an highly recommended to both laymen and professionals.

REVIEW
by Paul Shirley MSW, 7-17-2000

Kathi Stringer has taken on the difficulties of expressing human behavior in terms of one of the most abstract of psychological theories, which is object relations theory. Object relations theory is valuable to us for its unique ability to explain the subtle intricacies of thorny behavioral problems such as narcissism and borderline conditions. Object relations theory also has one distinct disadvantage, however, and that is the unfortunate fact that it is just very hard for concrete thinkers to understand it. To concrete thinkers, object relations theory often makes no sense at all: what are all those "internal objects," they want to know, and where are they?

How do we know they are even there? Can anyone "prove" to me that internal objects exist? The answer, unfortunately, is that there is no way to prove the existence of internal objects any more than it is possible to explain Victor Borge's incredible musical humor to non-musical persons. I actually tried doing that once, as a grad student. I found that trying to explain to non-musical persons that a classical chord sequence followed by a jazz resolution is somehow comical - well, it just doesn't work. The non-musical person just don't get it. Borge's kind of humor falls flat, even with an otherwise sharp person who is trying to be natural. (Sorry. No more puns.)

Kathi has brought several elements from different models together in a way that makes the inherent abstraction of the object relations theory easier to grasp. She has married one of the most complex "inward" looking psychological models, object relations theory, to a simpler and more "outward" looking sociological economic exchange type of theory. Then, she has combined those two disparate elements together into a visual transactional model which makes the whole thing appear elegantly simple. It also makes the abstract processes of object relations, especially the matter of projection, easy to visualize. The basics of transactional models are really as simple as kindergartners sharing toys: "You give me the doll, and I'll give you the ball." It's as simple a child's game, except that it's applied to feelings and thoughts. To me, though, the strongest point of Kathi's diagram is not its simplicity. The strongest point is that it compacts a great deal of complex, useful information in small space. I can see, for instance, Kathi's diagrams being eminently useful in the process of clinical supervision. In a nutshell, Kathi's work here is one example of the communicative power derived from combining an empirical social perspective with an hypothesized intra-psychic perspective. Kathi, not being burdened by professional psychological jargon, is apparently unaware that those two types of models don't normally go together, and so like the bumblebee that flies despite the scientific community's having proven that it cannot - Kathi's work flies too.

I appreciate the difficulties that some people have in grasping object relations theory, because I have a similarly hard time grasping abstract visual art. I mean even despite having taken a course in it, I still have a hard time with it. I just can't usually figure out what those wild colors, lines, triangles, circles, and weirdo shapes are all about. With the help of a good art instructor, though, I have had the pleasurable "aha" experience of standing in front of an abstract painting and suddenly feeling myself somehow in tune with the artist. (See? I had to resort to a musical metaphor!) Hopefully, Kathi's contribution on object relations will offer the same kind of thing, a psychological equivalent to my art instructor's showing me a glimpse of the inner world of abstract art. Object relations theory can open up astonishing whole new vistas of psychological understanding, and obviously Kathi Stringer keenly appreciates that fact. Kathi seems to share the same dream that drives artists to create, and that is the urge to share on the personal, emotional, and spiritual levels of experience. I for one appreciate her work and her values.

Now the Essay:

An Object Relations Approach to Understanding Projective Identification and Borderline Personality Disorder

Written by Kathi Stringer

The object of this discussion is to clarify and consummate the often confusing material written on the subject of Projective Identification and its concomitants. This model of object relations consists of three components. They are, Projective Identification, Projective Counter Identification and Introjective Identification. The three are interrelated and overlapped. The first two components are executed instantaneously by the unconscious from the interplay of transference / counter-transference.

To describe the dynamic of Projective Identification we must first establish the link between the patient and the treater. Within the patient resides the bad self, good self, good object and bad object. This leads to another process called, "splitting." A patient will split off repressed parts and project them onto the treater and then identify with treater. To be simplistic and to better suit our purposes we will use the paradigm of projecting the bad object from the patient into the treater albeit any object could be projected. The constellation of the bad object consists of the distorted cognition and maladaptive core beliefs of the patient usually caused from child abuse. When projecting the bad object the patient will elicit negative responses from the treater who provided a hook arousing the treater's counter-transference. One cannot project into a hollow shell. As individuals, we all carry with us the framework consisting of objects, an internal mental structure developed though out life.

When dealing with Borderline patents, countertransference is pervasive and must be continually reassessed in order for treatment to be efficacious. A treater applying an intervention asked a patient if he was aware that he was projecting his anger. The patient respond, "Can you think of anything better to do with it?"

> "I know when I am dealing with an abused child
> when I feel like strangling her myself."

Once this bad object has been projected and hooked by the treater, the treater then becomes the bad object. This component is known as Counter Projective Identification. The patient can now attempt to control the treater by manipulating the bad object enmeshed within the intrapsychic structure of the treater. As one therapist said, ***"I know when I am dealing with an abused child when I feel like strangling her myself."*** When a child is abused, she internalizes and incorporates this badness and will project it impulsively to elicit negative behavioral traits from the treater. This dynamic takes place instantly and unconsciously.

The critical component of this model is Introjective Identification. With counter-transference management, the treater can identify and contain the bad object, modify it, which is then reintorjected by the patient and assimilated. To illustrate this I will use the following example; A resident treating a contemptuous, defensive borderline patient was becoming extremely frustrated with her slanderous remarks. One day he was pushed over the line when she said, "I hope you don't quite your day job if you go into practice. I mean, look at the way you dress! You will never be able to attract clients!" Withdrawing from this interaction he reflected on this event and noticed that he was becoming just like the abusive patient. When he reproached her, he said, "I am trying to understand what is happening here. When I try and help you, you become abusive. I really want to help, don't you think we can work on this together?"

This response was unexpected by the patient. In this instance the treater identified and contained the bad object. When he respond with empathy, using coping strategies and aware of his impending countertransference, he modified her internal core beliefs. The treater also created a "holding environment, an empathic extension for the patient. It is important that this holding environment be consistent.

Obstreperous borderline patients are insecure in the world around them. They have concrete dysfunctional beliefs that they are bad, carrying with them the memories of child abuse. This impedes growth since they believe that they can destroy the good object and it will not survive. Incessantly testing limits, hoping for some sense of unmovable boundaries, they are often disappointed by destroying the all good object thereby preventing them from internalizing the goodness of society. All to often their behavior is mirrored back unempathicly reinforcing the empty-self, which substantiates their personal convictions. What they long for is the perfect caregiver who can accept their rage and idealizations and save them from the inadequate mother.

Too often the nurse and her contemporaries are ill advised or not sufficiently trained.

It would be unrealistic to believe that an affirmative omnipotent milieu exists. Yet, with structure and a carefully selected treatment plan, using alternate methods to preserve the good object, a borderline patient can assimilate her environment and redefined her beliefs. Nursing personal and treating staff must have a comprehensive knowledge of the fundamentals of mental mechanisms, adaptation styles, coping strategies and therapeutic intervention skills. This improved, goal oriented, therapeutic nurse-patient relationship and an understanding of communication skills, respect, desire to help will facilitate and redefine the borderline's interpersonal world. As one nurse said, "Kill the borderline's effect with kindness."

Too often the nurse and her contemporaries are ill advised or not sufficiently trained. This will diminished growth and reinforce the patient's intrinsic pessimistic beliefs. This manifests and invokes undesired behavior extrapolated from their interpersonal contact with the professional staff. The goal would be to validate the patient's traumatic past, yet focus on the here-and-now using interpretation as therapeutic tool. Validation is important to advance the alliance with the patient. All to often the treater will insist the this anger belongs to the patient and doesn't want it crammed down his throat. It would be therapeutically advantageous for the treater to contain the projected anger and hold it, again providing a holding environment.

It is my intent that this paper has illustrated the concept of Projective Identification as a useful instrument to agglomerate in the framework of object relations. Thank you for your interest.

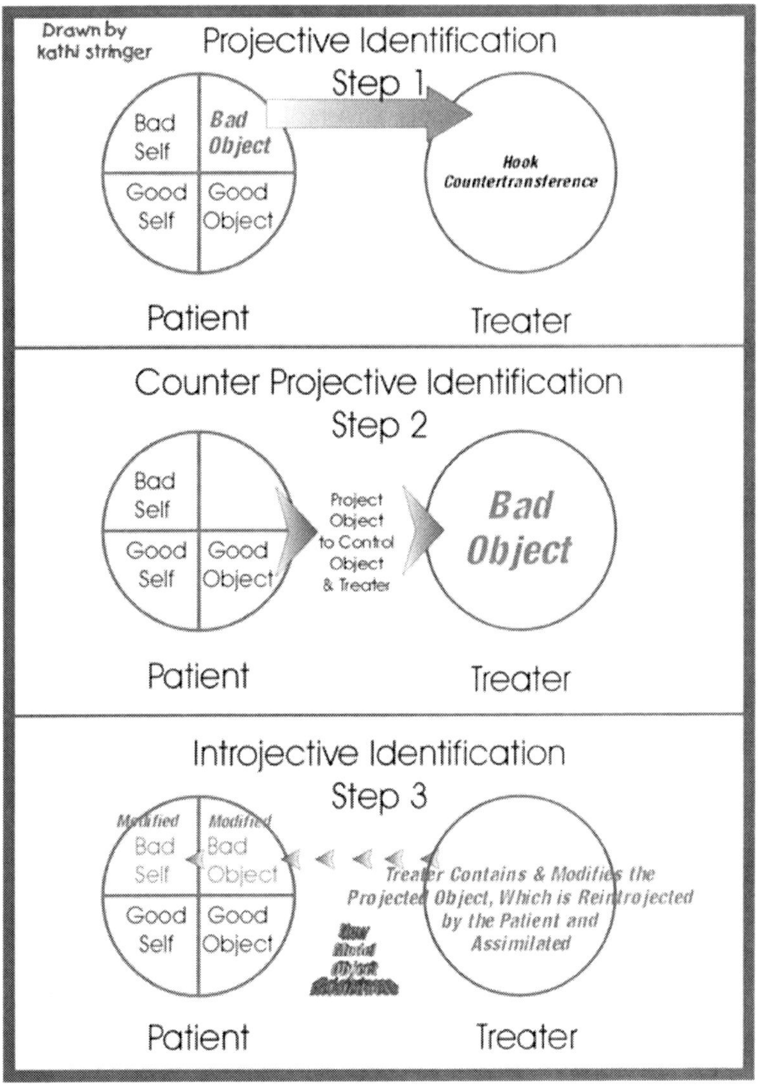
Drawn by kathi stringer
Projective Identification
Step 1
Bad Self
Bad Object
Good Self
Good Object
Hook
Countertransference
Patient
Treater
Counter Projective Identification
Step 2
Bad Self
Good Self
Good Object
Project Object to Control Object & Treater
Bad Object
Patient
Treater
Introjective Identification
Step 3
Modified Bad Self
Modified Bad Object
Good Self
Good Object
Treater Contains & Modifies the Projected Object, Which is Reintrojected by the Patient and Assimilated
Patient
Treater

Holding Environment for the Individual with Borderline Personality Disorder

Written by Kathi Stringer

With this discussion I hope to elaborate on the conceptualization and aesthetic fundamentals of the empathic holding environment when applied in the treatment of the borderline patient. When treating the borderline, the therapist is working with primitive defense mechanisms (spitting & projective identification covered earlier) in most lower level clients. To draw from an analogy, the best paradigm leads to the environment of the toddler. This would be a good place to begin since the first three years of life are crucial in the human development of how we relate to the world.

The newly ambulatory toddler struggles daily with the conflicting components of independence / individuality verses dependence / enmeshment with the primary caregiver. The toddler, testing limits in his expanding world retreats periodically to mother for emotional refueling. If the mother is unavailable in this critical phase, the toddler will be reluctant to develop his growing autonomy. Rather, he interprets the event of leaving mother as abandonment since on his return, she is unavailable. The toddler's response is clingy behavior. Yet, not to enlarge his budding world means engulfment by her.

The ambiguous thoughts of the toddler become overwhelming in the splitting format of independence verses dependence. Unable to articulate his thoughts and bridge both dynamics into a comprise, the toddler gives in to rage often seen as a temper tantrum. Unable to make a decision in his confusion, the parent would do well to hold the child. This would demonstrate to the child even in his rage, he cannot destroy the parent or the empathic holding environment provided for him. This then, leads to the emergence of a consistent constant object in his mental structure, which is similar to the (Erikson) theory of *trust* Vs *mistrust*. It is irrelevant the source of the frustration, real or imagined. The point is, it is real for the toddler and must be addressed as such. A parent that will provide a consistent empathic holding environment will pave the way for trust and object constancy (Winnicott).

The therapist's office, the milieu of a hospital setting, are sufficient to maintain this environment with the borderline patient. The borderline longs for the perfect caregiver. Patients may well come to feel that they are with someone who is strong enough to withstand their destructive impulses (Cohen & Sherwood) and interested enough to engage them even in their painful state. Since Adler and Buie believe that the core of the borderline pathology is a failure in the development of holding and soothing introjects, they argue that the early stages of therapy must offer patients the experience of being empathically held. Cohen and Sherwood (1996) go on to say, "The borderline will emphasize the therapist's coming to be seen as a stable, consistent, and caring person who survives the patient's rage." Like the toddler, the borderline will incessantly test limits hoping to find consistent boundaries.

Treatment Team Countertransference Awareness

Written by Kathi Stringer

An effective therapeutic alliance is supported on the foundation of the treatment team's countertransference awareness and management. If left unmonitored or unidentified, it can lead to staff burnout, resentment, and turnover. Certainly, a disturbing element is the drop in staff moral and emotional plasticity. The by-product of ineffective countertransference management from the team as a collective can lead to a "domino-effect" of patient's unresponsiveness and uncooperation.

These motivating factors from countertransference necessitate implications to consider the teams resources, skills, history and capacity to function synergistically and effectively. For example, perhaps staff had a difficult patient and the remnants of resentment or unresolved conflicts are still emotionally engaged and then 'transferred" to the new patient. As Paris (1993) states, "*The countertransference response may reflect unresolved issues in the team's history of working with a certain kind of patient.*" We see here how countertransference history is important and must be acknowledged. Equally important is the task of introducing and reviewing of new or contemporary therapeutic skills coupled with the teams resources. And finally, the team's capacity to therapeutically meet the treatment needs of the unit's caseload and demands. Any variation in the parameters of the teams resources, skills, history and capacity can dynamically affect countertransference reactions to the patients. In other words, depending on the measures of the above independent properties the team may react different countertransferentially to the patient population at any one time.

Keep Tools Sharp

As every successful and competitive industry acknowledges, one criteria is certain, and that is the tools of the trade must be continually be sharpened to keep from becoming dull. These savvy companies survive through savings or profits or a combination of both. Dull tools make for poor productivity. A sharp tool can boost effectiveness while cutting downtime. This will create dual pockets, one for profits and the other for savings. If mental health providers would give serious consideration to creating a position in the staff hierarchy, therapeutic tools would remain on the competitive edge.

This newly created position would belong to a full time facilitator and the duties would be similar to the duties of a patient group facilitator with the exception of being professionally targeted. The facilitator would bring in new ideas while mobilizing dull skills to the surface and reintegrating them into fresh creative methods.

This would boost the treatment team's spirit, moral and confidence towards themselves and the patient. Paris states, "*The treatment staff, both individually and collectively, need to feel that their therapeutic contributions are acknowledged, respected, and valued.*"

The Execution Boundary and Borderline Hatred

Written by Kathi Stringer

Special Thanks to Nicole for Inspiring Me to Write this Paper
The idea of writing this paper came up because after examining my own feelings and talking to individuals with borderline personality disorder, the issue seemed to come up frequently that their treater would threaten to ban them from the practice because of their primitive rage acted out in transference.

Topographical Model

The material in this paper is based on the modern psychodynamic psychotherapy model embedded in object relations.

Abandonment and Rejection

The execution boundary and abandonment are one of the same in the mind of a borderline. That said, before we discuss the execution boundary, lets reflect on the borderline's desperation to prevent separation and loss. Adler reflects the borderline wishes;

> "*Borderline patients talk vividly about their longings to be held and contained, and their panic about being dropped, abandoned and rejected* (p.221)."

> Searles echoes Adler, "*borderline personality-organization itself renders ever-present, for him, the danger of separation and loss* (p.288)"

This basic intrinsic borderline pathology and its destructive power will be the theme for this paper.

Using Transference in the Analytic Space

Since we are going to include transference in this discussion would be useful to review its basic fundamental significance.

Transference is feelings and attitudes from previous relationships of the past and brought into the present and directed toward the treater. Of course, transference is always a distortion but extremely useful to examine the internal structures of the borderline. Kernberg interprets transference in this way,

> “*Transference is usually conceptualized as the transfer of love or hatred from the original object onto the therapist* (p.156).”

For example a client may direct rage to the treater seen as the parental object since this rage is, in reality, rightfully at parents. Through this transference a client is able to work out this anger in the analytic space.

The analytic space is the realm where assigned roles are played out and examined to identify defenses and developmental organization of regressed individuals.

Reassignment of Ego Strength

A frighten mistrustful borderline may attempt to devalue the therapist and reassign the treater's ego as helpless, weak and insignificant. The unconscious dynamic that may play out is now the client is in the safe controlling role of parent, able to torment the child, aka the treater. To the borderline it gives a sense of being in a position of doing the rejecting instead of being rejected. The pseudo gain from the switch gives rise to the prominent idea that the treater cannot destroy the patient. Truly a paradox since most borderlines have infantile longings to be contained and nurtured and this exchange prevents exactly that.

Lets talk about the Countertransference Hook

I think it is important to briefly touch on countertransference for a moment to see how it plays into the execution boundary.

Countertransference is a term that describes a jointly created phenomenon between the treater and the client. In essence, countertransference is a reaction from the client's transference combined with the unconscious unresolved issues of the treater. For example lets say a client brings past unresolved anger from a previous relationship and projects it onto the therapist. When this projection of anger from the client is combined with pressure, as if to force the treater to behave in line with the clients wishes, we call this projective identification, since the client is identifying with the treater to project the object (anger). Think of it as a client unconsciously pushing the hot buttons of the treater, as if the client is taking her anger out on the treater. In order for the client to take her anger out on the treater and get the desired reaction, the treater must have some sort of weakness that is identified by the client. Once identified, this becomes a countertransference hook, a hot button, which of course can hook the treater to behave in such a way as the client is projecting. One cannot project into a hollow shell. Like a small child may think, “I made mommy do what I wanted her to do.”

I think it is important to describe the countertransference hook as it relates to anger projected from the client in transference from previous relationships. Perhaps if the treater were aware of the dynamic he would be able to detach and not take the projected anger as personal. Which is difficult since the projection was custom tailored for the treater as identified by the client via his ego weaknesses. With practice and hyper diligence the treater may be able to contain the projection without retaliating.

Projective Identification via the Hot Button

Some borderlines are so terrified of annihilation, of getting erased, of being thrown into the dark abyss that they will protect themselves by zeroing in on the countertransference hook of the treater.

Adler insightfully describes a borderlines fear;

> "*These patients are expert in perceiving aspects of the therapist's personality that are problem areas for the therapist. Primitive patients probably develop this skill from their style of existence, in which every encounter with any person is so threatening that they must perceive his weaknesses in order to be prepared for the final battle for survival* (p.180)"

Most borderlines seem to have a honing device that directs them to the therapist's ego weakness. Once this weakness is identified, a borderline may push the treater's hot buttons defined previously as a countertransference hook. Once the treater is hooked through projective identification, the client has now gained a sense of control, if and only if, the treater identifies with the projection. If the borderline is successful and the treater identifies with the projection, (anger in this case) then what we call projective counteridentification has taken place (Ogden 1982). In other words the treater now behaves characteristically similar to the internal drama of the borderline (Adler), as if an alien force has taken the treater over (Gabbard). Sometimes the projective counteridentification is so miserable for the treater that he may take this dilemma under consultation. Kernberg reminds us that,

> "*Under conditions of projective counteridentification the therapist may unreasonably feel unfit to treat the patient* (p. 86)."

Since the treater may feel unreasonably unfit to treat the patient, the treater may threaten the client with the execution boundary. However, in cases under supervision or by consultation, it is here where the opportunity of magic begins. The treater is now in a position to respond in a kinder way providing a new experience for the borderline to internalize. This is what we call an introject. The treater is now offering a positive introject to the borderline, and if accepted, it may be taken in and assimilated. This is referred to as introjective identification. Meaning the client has identified and accepted the new experience from the treater and is willing to take it in to be assimilated. The client is now able to see the world as a modified and newer place in which to live.

Advantage of Acting out Anger in Transference

A therapist that prevents regressive developmental behaviors (anger) from being examined in the analytic space can fixate or prolong therapy since the dynamic that drives the pattern cannot be identified in the transference. The threat of an execution boundary for vocally expressing anger may be interpreted as the ultimate abandonment and rejection; a devastating borderline injury. The alternative as Adler so eloquently states;

> "*The therapist's consistent, tactful, non-retaliatory handling of the patient's rage allows the pathological defenses to be given up slowly and permits the patient to experience the therapist as the truly good object who can safely be intorjected* (p176)."

> Gunderson also advocates the tolerance of negative transference as a basic tenet; "*The therapist must be able to withstand the borderline's verbal assaults without either retaliating or withdrawing. By this process, the patient's hostility can be examined and understood as part of a more general pattern of relating to important others.*"

The Holding Environment and Modified Introjects

The analytic space created in the therapeutic framework is what Winnicott (1965) referred to as the '*Holding Environment.*' This provides a safe environment for the borderline to establish trust in the treater as the good object. Applegate & Bonovitz suggest that;

> "*it is only when a sense of safety and trust finds solid footing in a secure clinical holding environment and ego relatedness with the clinician is established that clients can begin to risk testing the clinician's durability.*"

Once testing begins, consciously or unconsciously a treater can modify the projected hostilely and rage into a softer, soother objects and offer it back to the borderline as a modified positive introject. Apparently, since it took years to form the borderline personality, it will also take collaborative work, bit-by-bit, for the borderline to re-trust, relearn, and re-identify with something better then their terrifying internal objects. Some borderlines have burning determination to go back into the past via transference to the treater and resolve the anger that was emotionally fixated from an earlier period.

With most borderline personalities, trust is a funny thing. It reminds me of a tid-bit I remember that goes like this, "If the employee gets 1000 at-a-boys, then he shall receive the promotion as company president, but one ah-shit along the way, and the process starts all over again." It is frustrating to a treater to start over because of a countertransference reaction caught by a receptive hypersensitive borderline. Perhaps the treater may reduce the at-a-boys toward a successful conclusion of treatment if the execution boundary did not constantly raise it's ugly head and start the trusting process all over again.

Further exploration in some cases may reveal an unconscious narcissist longing in the treater, rooted in countertransference, to encourage dependency from the borderline. Since setting the execution boundary with regular reminders may cause a borderline to become clingier, more frantic, desperate, anxious, and distressed, then this would seem to satisfy the treaters unconscious wish for dependency. The problem is, this may hinder trust in the therapeutic alliance and of particular discern, treatment may be extended over a longer duration rising out of what a primitive personality may perceive as exclusion from the family relationship. "I am still bad and I can be cast out, and you have been lying to me all along that you really care about me. See, I knew this would happen."

Harmful Introjects

Most borderlines worst fears stem from abandonment and rejection ideation. This terrifying pathology drives them to unconsciously compare any interpretation, facial expression or gesture as clues to impending doom. This undifferentiatedness helps explain why the execution boundary acts as a cathexis to feed borderline fear and regressive behaviors, which causes at times resentment from the treater in the form of negative introjects. Searles adds,

> "*Much 'self'-destructive behavior on the patient's part consists in his having introjected some of this most primitive, "sickest" components of the analyst's ego-functioning and, in the acting out, venting aggression upon this introject* (p.323)."

This describes the effect a negative introject can have on a client in the form of self-destruction. The execution boundary tossed into the therapeutic arena may certainly be a countertransference reaction from the treater to punish the client. The problem is, words are powerful and especially powerful when assimilated by the client from an idealized treater.

The execution boundary is so powerful, so devastating, and so frightening, that the mere suggestion of it's essence can set back treatment for months.

A Paradox

So it seems we have a sort of paradox here. The treater perceives that setting the execution boundary will limit acting out in rage; however, this capital boundary may fixate progress, impede the development of trust and hinder the formation of a constant object. Ironically the very rage the treater intended to emotionally restrict manifests in the borderline's developmental defects giving rise to unwanted regressive symptoms. These regressive characteristics may take the form of dependency, neediness and self-destructive behavior since aggression is turn inward on self. On aggression, Catham explains,

> "*They have no way to modulate this aggression because they have not achieved the cognitive prerequisites for doing so* (p.197)."

In fundamental nature, setting a capital boundary to contain rage may also regress the borderlines internal structures leading to desperation.

Conclusion

The mere oppression of the execution boundary can manifest in the form of regressive defensives in the borderline and prolong or destroy therapy all together. The borderline may prematurely terminate therapy in anticipation of getting terminated. This should be of primary concern for treaters that wish expedient recovery for their borderline patients. I recall a saying that when like this, "Violence is the last resort of the incompetent" Execution or a creditable threat in the mind of a borderline is just as devastating

References:

1. Effective Psychotherapy with Borderline Patients / Waldinger & Gunderson [1989]
2. Countertransference and Regression / Boyer [1999]
3. Borderline Psychopathology and Its Treatment / Adler [1985]
4. The Facilitating Partnership / Applegate & Bonovitz [1995]
5. The Psychiatric Annals Volume 32, Number 6 [2002]
6. The Narcissistic and Borderline Disorders / Masterson [1981]

7. Psychodynamic Psychotherapy of Borderline Patients / Kernberg [1989]
8. Intensive Psychotherapy of the Borderline Patient / Chessick [1983]
9. Borderline Personality Disorder / Gunderson [1984]
10. Management of Countertransference with Borderline Patients / Gabbard [1994]
11. Treatment of Patients in the Borderline Spectrum / Meissner [1995]
12. Borderline Personality Disorder, A Clinical Guide / Gunderson [2001]
13. My Work with Borderline Patients / Searles [1990]
14. Countertransference Issues in Psychiatric Treatment / Gabbard [1999]
15. Psychodynamic Psychiatry in Clinical Practice DSM-IV Ed. / Gabbard [1994]
16. Treatment of the Borderline Personality / Chatham [1985]

On Empathy

First Responders

&

Inpatient

Cops, Cop-Out on Empathy?

Written by Kathi Stringer

Professional Feedback

CORONA POLICE DEPARTMENT

849 WEST SIXTH STREET (PO BOX 940) CORONA, CALIFORNIA 91718-0090

"Your research article titled "Cops, Cop-Out on Empathy?" was extremely informative and educational. Sgt. Rodriguez has already shared some of the material used in your article to provide additional training to the officers in the field. The feedback he received from the officers was well received."

- **Richard E. Madory**
Captain Field Services Division
Commander
Corona Police Department – Corona CA

"Thank you for your excellent article and for the good use you've made of my work. It's very gratifying to have made a contribution that helps others make contributions."
- Susan Schwartz Senstad
Family Therapist provided psychotherapy for over 20 years. She has trained many consultants, teachers and therapists as facilitators.

"Stupendous piece of work! Spreading it all over the place now!"
- Sam Vaknin Ph. D.
The author of Malignant Self Love: Narcissism Revisited and other mailing lists (c. 4000 members).

Cops, Cop-Out on Empathy?

by Kathi Stringer
April 16, 2003

A look at protective agencies that are becoming more and more devoid of empathy. Could it be their underlying weakness?

> *One Complaint Investigation Field Officer for the Corona Police Department asked the question, "What is empathy? Do you mean, "Can I picture myself handcuffed to a hospital bed and the pain of a needle entering into a gash? No, I can't. I've never been in that position, so how could I possibly imagine that?"*

His response can boggle the mind of even those that have never been there before. It would seem reasonable to construct pieces of life's experiences to appreciate a close approximately of what it must be like to be trapped and in pain.

Scope:
This work is written in three parts:
1. Overview of Empathy
2. Empathy in Depth
3. Empathy, First Responders, Policemen and Firefighters

I. Overview of Empathy

What is Empathy?

The complex definition: Infopedia describes empathy this way:
*The imaginative projection of a subjective state into an object so that the object appears to be infused with it...*To say it another way, in the example above, "*The subjective feeling of pain from the victim, into the police officer, so that the police officer appears to have a understanding of the victims pain.*" To simplify it again, "*Understand the feelings of others, as you would have them understand your feelings.*" To say it again in Basic English: "I'm hurting! Please help me!"

The straightforward definition: Lauren Wispe (1991, p.80) describes empathy this way:

- In empathy the self is the vehicle for understanding, and it never loses its identity.
- In empathy one substitutes oneself for the other person.
- To know what something would be like for the other person is empathy.
- In empathy one acts "as if" one were the other person.
- The object of empathy is understanding.
- In sum, empathy is a way of knowing.

Most of us have never been confronted with "Sophie's Choice", a Mother and a German Jew that was faced with a heart-wrenching predicament. A German S.S. war criminal "*Ordered her to select one of her children, who would then be sent to the ovens; the other would be spared. This sequence is especially heartbreaking, as the screaming little girl is carried away to die.*" Even though this has not happened to most of us, we can appreciate the torment and agony of such a situation. ***We call this empathy***.

Basically, empathy is the *taking on the trial mind-set of another individual, to put one in the other person's shoes, without losing a sense of self.* For example: One asks, "Why is defending a rag, a piece of material so important?" The answer is symbolic, "because this material is the American Flag, and represents to many, the sacrifices made for freedom." This is particularly useful because one can predict with a measure of accuracy the consequences of burning the American Flag in a hostile environment of mothers and fathers that have lost their sons and daughters to a war. One must be empathetic to appreciate their losses and avoid the consequences.

What is Evil?

During the Nuremberg trials (from the holocaust), a U.S. Army Psychiatrist, Capt. Gilbert, (a Jew), routinely interviewed and built relationships with the Nazi war criminals. At the conclusion of the trail he discovered they all had a single common dominator. He stated, "***Evil is a lack of empathy, a total incapacity to feel with their fellow man.***" And Hart added, "***I would suggest that evil acts stem from a lack of empathy.***"

History Lesson and the Significant of Empathy

In the aftermath, decades later Governor Wilson budget included $2 million for the California Commission of Peace Offices Standards and Training to send 7,000 peace officers through a Law Enforcement ***Tools for Tolerance*** program at the Simon Wiesenthal Center's Museum of Tolerance in Los Angeles. The idea was to display the holocaust and the horror of hate crimes.

A Showcase of Empathy

The hit T.V. series, The Pretender, showed us a child prodigy, Jared, that was kidnap by a austere, foreboding and powerful agency known as The Centre. The Centre exploited Jared's genius through the development of SIMS, short for Simulations. Jared was given a set of parameters for targeted environments to enable him to process the probable outcome. Unknown to Jared, the Centre used his genius, his outcome of SIMS, to assassinate or massacre people. Strangely enough, the writer of the series did not appear to suggest that the crucial element of Jared's genius was his ability to empathize with others in order to determine their likely actions through SIMS. Without insight to empathy Jared could not have built complex analogies and assessed the percentages of likely outcomes.

Empathy as a Simulation

Nichols remarked that "Goldman's simulation alternative claimed that we understand others by simulating them in a way that produces empathy. Empathy always involves simulation, but may simultaneously include theory application." By properly specifying the processes of empathy, we are able to show the amount of theory needed to generate an accurate simulation.

On Sympathy:

Sympathy is feeling sorry for the individual. Nguyen states, "The big difference between the word "empathy" and its synonym "awareness" is that the sympathy is incorporated into the meaning of the word "empathy. Empathic people are those who express their feelings toward your problems with sympathy and understanding." A world devoid of insensitivity, indifference, and empathy to others' agony and suffering will, Nguyen says "end up being in a robot world where people live without any feeling." Sympathy lends to pitying and feeling sorry for a person. Empathy takes a solution-based stance to understand and solve the problem. Empathy is taking on the trail mindset of another individual, (through awareness or training) while maintaining ones personal sense-of-self, and the product is a jointly built communication that, (1) May develop into a warm personal regard, and / or (2) De-escalate a dangerous environment.

Scientific Measurement of Empathy

Empathy is always a simulation but it is possible to include theory-application to identify the sensation of empathy. At this time it is scientifically impossible to measure the accuracy of one's ability to successfully take on the trial mindset of another. What may appear humorous to one person may appear as horror to another in the extreme.

However, *awareness* of cultural norms, *awareness* of *typical* reactions to trauma, *awareness* of a range of appropriate emotions, can *help improve the percentages* of the measurement of empathy. For example, not every American will feel an allegiance to the American Flag, but though life's lessons one may avoid severe consequences of destroying this symbolic piece of material in precarious situations.

Acquiring Empathy, the Construct

Barnes & Thagard surmise that Empathy can be constructed though the use of analogy. *"Empathy can be difficult to achieve for some individuals but not impossible."* To acquire empathy one must be able to navigate though the mapping on one's personal experience (and willing) and relate it to the empathee. If one's personal experience is incomplete, then one must be able to actually draw a conjecture to understand and appreciate the empathee's situation through imagination.

> For example: The empathee appeared crestfallen, depressed, hopeless and isolative. To acquire empathy one would have to take on the trial mindset of the empathee. One would have to; (1) recall vividly the emotion of depression, i.e. – the loss of a loved one, and (2) recall the emotion of hopelessness, i.e. – the inability to solve a problem at one time, and (3) feeling or notion to run away from life's problems, i.e. – the desire to isolate. The willingness and desire to understand, to become ***aware***, are the parameters and properties of empathy.

Empathy Can Be a Tool

For those individuals in sales. If a sales person is able to identify with the buyer with empathy toward their problems (home, work, relationships), the sales agent is more likely to overcome the buyer's objections and offer applicable solutions based on the buyer's frame of mind. This works in three ways.

1. The Sales individual was able to put himself in the buyer's shoes to *understand his problems,* and
2. The sales individual was able to keep his own identity for problem solving and not get swallowed up into the buyer's misery so he could maintain an objective to solve the problem, and,
3. The final product that was attractive to the buyer was the joint collaboration, the joint communication that resonated though empathy. The use of empathy was the vehicle that initially developed trust to build the sales-to-buyer relationship.

An experienced sales agent will look for verbal and non-verbal clues to measure the strength and development of empathy as the conversation progresses. Hopefully the end result will be a win-win between the sales agent and the buyer. We call this *insight to empathy.*

On the flip side of 'insight to empathy,' the Nazi's were able to take on the trial mind-set of their enemies to terrorize them. They configured bombs with sirens, and as the bombs approached the target, the whistle of the sirens created panic. Empathy in this case was psychological warfare to terrify their victims.

II. Empathy In Depth

The Argument of "Empathy vs. Truth" – "Subjective vs. Objective"

Truth and Reality co-exist and are equivalent. Reality is Truth. Life experience taught us to arrive at the truth more quickly, and to separate the objective of reality from the subjective of fantasy. Dr. Vaknin quotes Morris, "*Closely related to the ability to read other people's emotions is* **empathy** *– the arousal of emotion in an observer that is a vicarious response to the other person's situation… Empathy depends not only on one's ability to identify someone else's emotions but also on one's capacity to put oneself in the other person's place and to experience an appropriate emotional response.*" Vaknin continued, " *Thus empathy does require the communication of feelings AND an agreement on the appropriate outcome of the communicated emotions. In the absence of such an agreement, we are faced with inappropriate affect (laughing at a funeral, for instance).*" In essence, those individuals that have ***experienced*** life more completely will be able to relate to the truth more quickly, and thus be more empathetic.

Experiencing Empathy

Vaknin states, "Empathy has little to do with the other person (the empathee). It is simply the result of conditioning and socialization. In other words, when we hurt someone - we don't experience his or her pain. We experience OUR pain. Hurting somebody hurts US. The reaction to pain is provoked in US by OUR own actions." Whether we choose to feel our pain or to block it out is a matter of choice. Vaknin raises some interesting questions. If we choose not to experience our pain, if we choose not to be vulnerable, then are we selfish and evil as the U.S. Army Psychiatrist Capt. Gilbert stated, "Evil is a lack of empathy, a total incapacity to feel with their fellow man?"

It certainly makes one wonder if it is possible to be civilized and also be devoid of empathy. Without empathy perhaps the world would be reduced to prey slaughtering prey. Eat or be eaten.

We have learned a lot about empathy since the Nuremberg trials. We have learned that empathy can manifest as good or evil. Good would be the genuine and authentic concern for the empthee. Evil would take on the trail mind set of the victim to identify, examine manipulate and annihilate the target.

A look at the Ego, Empathy and Training

The ego is the executive agency of the mind and makes the decision based on three sources (pressures) of information. To simplify, they are (1) pleasure seeking (impulsive) and the aspects needed to survive, (2) morals and perfection, formed out of punishment and rewards, and (3) the external world (reality). It is the Ego's function to reach a compromise between these three opposing forces, and to make a decision that is reality based.

> *Vaknin states: "Empathy is an internal reaction, an internal process, triggered by external cues...." Since empathy is an internal reaction (based on external in internal stimuli) then the perception of reality (truth) of the empathor is equally governed by the same rules and systems of the Ego (internal process based on external and internal stimuli). Now we can conjecture that empathy is directly hardwired to the Ego.*

There are massive volumes of scholarly material that attempt to explain the development and structures of the Ego, an individual's ability to relate to reality (truth) accurately, successfully and timely. To measure the ego would equate to measurement of empathy.

Vaknin suggests that empathy, or lack of it, is directly related to the individual's morals, cultural anthropology, especially with respect to social structure, and self-awareness. Since the Empathy is hardwired into the Ego, we can say that the function of the ego operates through thinking and reasoning which must negotiate between the psychosocial demands of reality and the demands of the self, and then comprise. The ego is also formed out of punishments and rewards that shape 'morals'. I draw this parallel to demonstrate that the Executive of the Ego, and Empathy are carried out in much the same way.

In other words, an individual is as assessable to his Ego and he is to his Empathy. Both are carried out as a 'reaction' or a 'response.' Both are shaped by life's experience. Both are shaped by genetics, temperament, and the synthesis of the mind meeting reality (truth). However, empathy operates out of the executive agency of the Ego. This gives us the choice as humans to develop (train) our empathy to be more in line with reality. In easy speak; an evil person is less likely to have *positive empathy* then most of us. We could say that person's personality (ego) is directly related to his or her understanding of relating to others with positive empathy.

Percentages

Vaknin reminds us that our personal inter-subjective (what we think) world may be completely different and out-of-sync with the inter-subjective (what they think) world empthee, and in such cases would render empathy meaningless. However, though clues, ego development, the desire to understand, and the desire to development a warm personal regard, we can immensely improve the percentages of the success of empathy.

III. Empathy, First Responders, Policemen and Firefighters

Positive Empathy, Attunement and Defense.

It could be argued that the restriction of empathy acts as a defense. For example: A police officer that has intervened in domestic abuse, that has responded to a rape call, that has interceded at a violent gang party, is hardly going to go home and select "Sophie's Choice" for the evening movie. It is likely at this point there would be an avoidance of empathy. Ochberg sums it up this way, "*We have not been directly exposed to the trauma scene, but we hear the story told with such intensity, or we hear similar stories so often, or we have the gift and curse of extreme empathy we suffer. We feel the feelings of our clients. We experience their fears. We dream their dreams. Eventually, we lose a certain spark of optimism, humor and hope. We tire. We aren't sick, but we aren't ourselves.*"

Protective agencies that have been spit on, beat on, and screamed at, may find it difficult to flip the empathy switch from one dispatch call to the next. Some agency employees that are burned out flip the empathy switch to 'off' as a protective maneuver, because to feel for others is draining and, quite frankly, the are spent. Other agency employees adjust their positive attunement to empathy lower then what would be normally expected to filter out the bulk of their stress. However, the question begs to be asked, "When does a professional create more harm then good because their positive attunement to empathy has failed the victim?"

Empathy as a Gage

Here, we go back to Wispe's description of empathy, "*In empathy the self is the vehicle for understanding, and it never loses its identity.*" This is important. ***Empathy is a tool, a gage, and a barometer to assist the professional to help the victim. It does NOT mean the professional should own the feelings of the victim.*** If the professional were to cross-the-line, sort of speak, and OWN the feelings of the victim, then it is likely that the professional would feel miserable, depressed, and ineffective. Using empathy appropriately, the professional can respond to ease grief, sadness, invalidation and trauma. Empathy conveys awareness, an attunement to the victim. For example, to withhold empathy can stir feelings of "*Rage at injustice and stupidity and people who treat him as less than he is.*" One father of a victim said, "*It is not every day that we see protective* *agencies that care enough to look at us as human beings, not just a situation. That would take empathy."*

Empathy and Vulnerability

Police, Firefighters, First Responders and other protective agencies are usually guarded with a wall of *in*vulnerability that seems to be inherent of their position. *In*vulnerability is viewed as strength while vulnerability is viewed as flawed and weak. This wall-off stance against vulnerability is problematic toward empathy as Susan Senstad states, "*When we are able to feel our vulnerability, we are able to experience the full range of our emotions to the world around us*" and "*Vulnerability is the unique capacity for receptivity and empathy which allows human beings to acknowledge and care for their ethical responsibility for each other, for the community and their environment.*" In other words, the wall of *in*vulnerability can prevent empathy and re-traumatize the individual with the *trauma of treatment*.

> Senstad recalls her unreachable father in her words: "*Daddy is a lot like God", my sister and I used to say, "Except that God is easier to make contact with." Daddy presented himself as strong, self-assured, decisive – and totally invulnerable.*

The difficulty with our society and culture is that it appears to present a no-win for protective agencies. Many individuals as Senstad expressed "*seemed to be far more attached to the myth of agencies omnipotence, and far more active in imprisoning them in that myth, then anyone would dare realize.*" Senstad continued, "*The fact that vulnerability may be a positive thing which requires openness does not mean, however, that people would do well go around without any armor.*" This armor impedes empathy, and the feelings of "wounds from losses, fears, shocks, humiliations, failures abandonments – the emotional baggage we carry from childhood." However, it is an axiom that "***Without access to vulnerability we lack the capacity for empathy***, and to develop our own sense of ethics. ***If we don't have access to our vulnerability, every encounter becomes a power-play, a struggle over control and status."***

Example: An attempted suicide victim was brought to Corona Regional Medical Center to be treated for a large gash on her wrist. When she flinched from the needle entering into her wound, a Corona Police Officer slammed down on a handcuff to subdue the victim with pain in order to contain the situation. The victim however, began trashing about from the apparent severe lack of empathy from this Police Officer. When the victim screamed at the police officer for his evident lack of empathy, and requested the office to readjust the handcuff, he refused. What happened? The Police Officer could have acted out of reaction to contain the situation, but then after he composed himself it would have been nice if he apologized. That did not happen. As Senstad implies, this Officer's complete lack of empathy invited a power play.

Senstad discovered a survivor in her research:

Helen Bamberg, who started The Medical Center for the Care of Victims of Torture in London and how, herself, survived the concentration camp at Bergen-Belsen, tells how the helpers who cared for liberated camp prisoners did just fine, Until, that is, the freed prisoners got stronger, started having opinions of their own, and what's more, started challenging the staff's authority. That made the helper anxious ergo furious; they'd lost their monopoly on strength.

It is a myth that in order for these protective agencies to be strong, the public must be vulnerable. This notion invites a one-up (agency), one-down (public), environment at first contact. Perhaps this police officer fed off the victim's vulnerabilities.

The lack of vulnerability and empathy in protective agencies may be due to deficient in-service training, staff turnover and burnout. Basically, those that are employed to 'serve and protect' have seen everything that can be seen, and their walls are firmly erected, and the public has become objects to be manipulated, contained, and dealt with.

Empathy as a Tool for De-escalation

The Houston Crisis Intervention Team reports:

Upon arriving at the scene, Officer Chillis found the individual depressed, very paranoid, and intent on taking his life. Initially, it was difficult to communicate with him. Officer Chillis gave the man plenty of space, allowed him to ventilate, actively listened, was patient, ***showed empathy*** and concern, and took a non-threatening stance. What appeared to be especially effective, Chillis said, ***was the use of body language to demonstrate a true concern and empathy*** for the confrontational demeanor helped convince the individual that Officer Chillis care about him and was there to help. The techniques worked. The individual opened up to Officer Chillis and talked to her about his personal problems that led to his depression. Officer Chillis credits the CIT training with providing skills that her de-escalate this situation.

Officer Chillis was able to save a life because she used empathy as a tool, a gage, to **become aware**.

Trauma of Treatment (First Contact)

"*Secondary wounding experience can be as painful and powerful as the original traumatic event,*" said Dr. Matsakis from her book titled, "I can't get over it," a hand-book for trauma survivors. She insightfully validated her readers that, "*You need to learn that, generally, the rejection, the humiliation, or attack says more about the ignorance, insensitivity, fears, or prejudices of the other person than anything about you, and that it reflects larger societal problems."*

There are times when the actual treatment (first contact) is as traumatic as the actual trauma itself. For example: In the case of the Police Officer, hammering down on the handcuff when the victim flinched in pain validated the original trauma in the victim's mind and that she deserved the childhood beatings from the past (PTSD). The victim felt as though an alien on the wrong planet and that her own kind would not have treated her this way. However, empathy, and a warm positive regard could have prevented the trauma -of –treatment. Since the Police Officer appeared devoid of empathy, his contact was harmful.

Intent

Most Police, First Responders, and Firefighters hope their position would help the victims and improve lives. Perhaps their heart is in the right place, but many are *unaware*. It would be tragic to respond with the intention of saving a life, and then have all that energy wasted because it did more harm then good, but it happens frequently from lack of empathy.

Summery

1. Empathy is taking on the trail mindset of the victim <u>without</u> losing a sense of self.

2. Empathy can be a valuable tool, a gage to de-escalate the situation

3. History has taught a lesson on the importance of empathy

4. Empathy can prevent the 'trauma of treatment"

5. The percentages of the attunement of empathy is directly related to the individual's willingness to become AWARE

6. Empathy is strength based, not a weakness

7. Empathy can save lives.

Recommendations:

(1) Perhaps this document may be helpful to protective agencies. Complimentary use is encouraged. (2) Create an environment, and a climate, to promote awareness (empathy). This may be accomplished through education and a desire to understand. It would be especially helpful if victims were invited to speak before First Responders, Police and

Firefighters to put a face behind the trauma. As one person said, "*I want to break down the barrier that creates an "us-versus-them" attitude into a "we-are-going-to-get-through-this-crisis-together" team approach.*"

Epilog

My personal hurt and pain inspired me to write this paper. I was the individual on that hospital bed when the Police Officer slammed down on the handcuff while the physician assistant applied twenty-one stitches. It is my sincere hope that this work might bring insight to *understanding empathy; the ability to become aware*.

References:

On Empathy
Sam Vaknin, Ph.D.
http://www.toddlertime.com/sam/empathy.htm

Essay on Empathy
Nguyen Minh Hien,
http://www.cs.uwm.edu/~nguyen/writings/sensitivity.htm

Houston Crisis Intervention Team
http://www.ci.houston.tx.us/departme/police/cit15.htm

The Wisdom of Vulnerability
Susan Schwartz Senstad
http://www.delos-inc.com/Reading_Room/
Articles/18/18.html

Empathy and Analogy
Allison Barnes and Paul Thagard
http://cogsci.uwaterloo.ca/Articles/Pages/Empathy.html

Mindreading and the Cognitive Architecture
underlying Altruistic Motivation
Shaun Nichols
http://www.cofc.edu/~nichols/cogaltFINAL.htm

Judicial Racism?
Roger Ivan Hart

Sophie's Choice.
James Stolee
http://www.mindspring.com/~lychelle/movies/sophies.htm

Tramua
Frank Ochberg MD

I Can't Get Over It
Aphrodite Matsakis, Ph.D.

Tabitha

Written by Kathi Stringer

Tabitha. I remember her fondly and have decided to share a bit of Tabitha with the world. We met as inpatients at the Adventist Medical Center in Portland Oregon. We were both diagnosed with borderline personality disorder. I guess I bring this up since some professionals have a hard time working with this group of individuals. So anyway, lets get on with meeting the lil girl in a hard world.

Tabitha, she was a tough girl at nineteen. She had rosy cheeks. Not because they were naturally rosy but because she continuously scratched them until they looked liked the scuffed knee of a toddler. With dark hair that framed her somewhat childish face, she put on the front of being every bit the hard-hitting girl.

We out hung out in the main room and watched television, all the while exchanging our criticisms of staff, cracking jokes and engaging in friendly discussions to get beyond the dull void of boredom.

As I got to know Tabitha a bit better, I felt a nature of protectiveness toward her. She was the abandon child. There were no visitors for her. Old clothes, leftovers from previous patients hung on her small figure. Overt in her topics, she concealed the love-starved child within under a masque that she herself was unable to penetrate.

Even though I was hospitalized to work on my own issues, I couldn't help but gravitate toward this despairing child. I guess, it was a reflection of myself, and helping Tabitha would in someway bring a new experience for myself vicariously through her.

As an attitude of off-the-cuff humor developed between us, there was also something else going on. A sort of bonding since I truly was hoping to find clues on how I may be able to help Tabitha. I recall the first time I actually asked her a serious question. It was something to do with family relationships or past abuse. She was silent and speechless. I think it was more from a lack of words to communicate feelings. She looked puzzled as she smiled and blew off the question in trade more comfortable topics.

Out of the blue one day she came looking for me. I was reading a book as she tapped me on the shoulder.

"Kathi, I'm going to call my mom. Do you want to come along and listen?" she asked with hope in her hazel eyes. It came to me just then that this was Tabitha's way of communicating her feelings that were lost in words and could not be said directly. I picked up on her cue.

"Sure Tabitha, I'll hang with you while you talk to your mom." I said. I felt like maybe I was able to make that nurturing connection that she seemed so desperately to be searching for. Perhaps, it was unexpected anyone could take an unselfish personal regard for her. I can't help it. My heart goes out of these individuals with bpd that are fixated in earlier developmental stages and are pledged with a parental emptiness. Maybe I could help fill her estranged abyss with a tiny fragment of human kindness unprovoked in the guise of a professional or predator. It's the best kind.

As she talked to her mother, it didn't take long to get the picture. Invalidation. Tabitha was being blamed for her hospitalization. As she protested, her tone turned to a sad and hopeless frustration. It was her fault. She deserved to be alone without visitors or clothes. She tearfully brought up her sexual abuse by extended family. It was nothing her mother hadn't heard before, and perhaps it was Tabitha's way to tell me her story. As she talked with her mother, I was attentive and focused. I wanted to be a witness for her sadness. It came to me just then why Tabitha scuffed up her delicate skin on her facial features. She was hurting, and this was the only way she knew of to show her pain. Poor thing. I wanted to scoop her up and take all her hurts away. But, I couldn't do that. Yet, I recalled through reading that offering a new experience could help change the world for a survivor. She was certainly that.

Later that day my friend Pat called and asked me if I needed him to bring anything during visiting hours. Gosh, how lucky I felt just then. My friends Pat and Trish came to visit me every day, and here was this lonely child putting on a tough appearance without anyone to ask if she needed or wanted anything. Just then an idea occurred to me. "Pat, hold on a second." Then I turned my attention to Tabitha. "Her Girl" I shouted, "Do you want my friends to bring you anything from the store?" Her eyes got big and round as she scanted a bit closer. "Can I have some of those rollo butterscotch and cherry candies?"

"Sure you can…anything else? How about a magazine? How about anything you want? Do you like M&M's?"

She smiled and nodded as if not exactly sure how to handle this. As she turned her attention away, I whispered to Pat, "Don't just get one bag of rollo butterscotch, get 10 bags of them and 10 bags of cherry ones too! And, pickup the National Enquire and the Reader's Digest and some teen magazines. Plus, find the biggest bag you can get of M&M's and get several of them. Also, get her a soother for comfort and some lifesavers." Back came a question from Pat, "How many lifesavers?" With laughter I said, "I don't know Pat, but make it a bunch. Impress me!"

As the day lingered on, Tabitha kept inquiring when Pat and Trish were going to show up. For a girl who seemed uninterested in getting anything, she sure showed plenty of interest. Of course, she had no idea whatsoever what was coming down the pike later that evening.

Tic-tock. Time drifted by we hung out in the main room. It was quite comfortable with several sofas encircling a table filled with torn magazines and cups half full of apple juice. Tabitha was sitting on the sofa with her knees up to her chest. Another patient was sprawled over an oversized chair with his feet dangling over the side. Some patients were talking just for the sake of talking, anything to breakup the boredom.

Then the visitors began to arrive. After awhile there was a lull in incoming visitors which prompt Tabitha to look at me exquisitely. Just then to familiar figures were coming down from the far end of the hall. It was Pat and Trish. They both looked quite funny loaded down with bags in each hand as they walked from side-to-side to maintain all the weight. Tabitha perked right up. "Hey girl" I said, "Your candy is here, and all the bags are for you. Go and see what ya got!" Pat and Trish flung the bags up onto the nurse's counter. Tabitha bopped over and then froze, as in terror. She did not expect this.

Oh my gosh, I thought. Tabitha appeared to be overwhelmed. She ran back to the main room away from the nurse's station. I sensed something. It was awkward. Tabitha was at a loss. I feared that maybe this may of hurt her, more then it helped. But no, it looked more like she did not experience this sort of friendship from anyone the way she cowered down. This vibrant tough kid was completely broken down. Her vocabulary that had been developed with a spark of "I'm big" became small as she peered back from the main room. I decided to redirect the attention off her and visit Pat and Trish so that perhaps she may find relief.

We had a good visit. My friends showing up like that reminded me how fortunate I was. I had friends to listen and believe me. I had friends to ally with me in support of my feelings. I was indeed very lucky. Friends of this sort enabled me to share with others. They give so much that it overflows from me to forgotten kids like Tabitha.

Pat and Trish already gone and I settled down to reading a book. Tabitha finally couldn't help herself and bopped back up to the nurse's station to claim her candy. Staff was a bit miffed and was wondering if I violated regulations. They clearly couldn't take this away from her. Not this child who was already deprived of visitors and wearing misfit clothing. Not her.

No matter about staff reluctance of my indulgence for Tabitha. I was determined that this little 'bad-kid' have an experience she could walk away with. An experience to reach down into her closed system of the starved invalidated child and offer up a small fragment of goodness from humanity. Possibly it may be what it takes to keep her alive at times. That the world can be a good place if we are lucky enough of find that special sort of love. The unconditional love from others without strings attached. Tabitha soon moved up a level as I rooted for her, encouraged her. She wanted to hang back with me, but I would have none of that. She needed to move on, and she did. It is somehow satisfying that when I think of the 'tough-girl', that she had a vestige of comfort to soothe her frighten and invalidated inner child. She got to see a bit of you and me reaching out in spirit, reaching out in life, reaching out in love. Tabitha saw a part of her mirrored back affectionately and was able to experience the greatest love of all, to love oneself. You go girl!

Stigma

and

Mental Illness

Stigma Meets Its Match

Written by Kathi Stringer

It was a cloudy day as the silver bird emerged from the clouds into a flight pattern. The aviator flipped the switches to prepare for landing. He checked his altimeter, leveled out the machine and touched down after a smooth decent. It was a perfect landing. The engine sputtered as he taxied down the runway. With experience and ease the aviator manipulated the rudders until the plane swung next to a hatch.

This story took place in a small peaceful town. Most of the residents knew each other on a first name basis. However, that day there was a problem. The sheriff responded to a call concerning a vagrant loitering on a city bench. He had seen his kind before on routine patrol. On occasion his task was clear up the bothersome vagrants when they appeared. The city just didn't put up with the unsightly trash and his job was to keep the city safe.

The man looked disheveled and worn. His face sprouted wiry hairs in contrast to his sunken eyes. It appeared he was dazed or perhaps lost in thought. Either way, he looked impaired and that made him dangerous. He had to go.

The law inquired as to the identity of the demented. He responded, "Howard, my name is Howard Hughes." The sheriff chucked, "Yeah right, I'm the Easter Bunny." He opened the rear door of the squad car and ran him in. The man continued his resolve as to this identity. It wasn't going to well. He must be drug addict or completely psychotic. The man was put behind bars to keep the town safe.

A few hours later a sheriff's friend rang his office for a friendly chat. In passing the sheriff rolled his eyes and said, "You won't believe who I have here today, Howard Hughes." It was a good chuckle for both of them. On the uptake his friend thought he might have a look at the stranger anyway. I mean after all, he was the junior vise president for a small satellite division of Hughes Aircraft, which was the main employer in town. It should be entertaining regardless.

Art Kemper, the Hughes executive arrived. Nicely groomed and professionally dressed, he looked at what appeared to be a homeless nobody. His wrinkled clothes matched the man's foul appearance. Art introduced himself as a Hughes Aircraft executive and the inquired as to his name. The lost soul glanced up from this bunk and replied, "I'm Howard Hughes." Art admitted he had never seen Howard Hughes before, but he did have one additional question that would clear things up. Art humorously asked, "Well now Howard Hughes, that is if you are really Howard Hughes that is, who do I work for? The vagrant's eyes became focused and steely as he replied, "You work for Dan Ferguson, and Dan Ferguson works for Hal Thomas, and Hal Thomas works for Ed Mason, and Ed Mason works for Noah Dietrich, and Noah Dietrich works for me." The sheriff grinned as he turned to look at Art. However, Art was not smiling. Something looked wrong. He looked financially terrified in response to stranger's reply. The words did not come as his eyes motioned to the sheriff there may be hell to pay. "My God Mr. Hughes," said Art in all sincerity. "It was an oversight. I'm so sorry! Sheriff, you had better let this man out of jail. If he wanted to, he could lay this whole town to waste with the flick of a pen." Stunned, the sheriff was stunned.

The vagrant climbed into his plane and with the turn of the switch power surged into the engine. He was Howard Hughes, a record-breaking aviator, inventor, playboy and billionaire. He was one of us.

The Quandary of Mental Illness as Stigma

Written by Kathi Stringer

Can the phrase 'mental illness' be de-stigmatized? We have seen the natural progression that "mental illness" equates to "mental sickness," and sickness when associated with 'mental' is instantly stigmatized and can immediately become an insult, "Man, you are one SICK puppy!" Now we see the dilemma, how can the mentally ill distance themselves from "the SICK puppies?" They can't. Not until they distance themselves from the word "sick." History offers an import lesson on this futile effort. Before I discuss this further, let us examine the natural flow of the early generational views of language as the decades sailed by.

Idiot. What if people began wearing a button that said, "Stop the stigma of being an Idiot?" And, what if there was a massive organized movement that exposed the film industry and contemporary literature as agents that are stigmatizing the mentally challenged individual with the inappropriate use of "idiot" as a demeaning adjective? Suppose the mission of the organization was to de-stigmatize the idiot, the imbecile and the moron. Do you think a movement like this could be successful? Could 'idiot' be clarified and resigned it's original meaning without insulting the mentally challenged with a renewed association that was lost over time? Further, would be possible that the mentally challenged and their loved ones would embrace such a crusade? Or rather, it would be likely they would try and put distance between the word and its meaning? Before answering these questions, lets examine the formation of stigma.

In 1940 it was proper to refer to the "mental deficient" as the idiot, the imbecile and the moron. A textbook titled "Psychiatry for Nurses" by Karnosh and Gage (1940) carefully instructs the student the correct classifications that have evolved into today's insult. Below is a direct quote from *Psychiatry of Nurses* (1940 - p. 237.)

> "Types of Mental Deficiency
>
> Idiot
> The *idiot* is one whose mental capacity is below the third-year level; they are clumsy, awkward, untidy and require constant supervision in the performance of the simplest requirement of living. Most idiots learn a few simple words but rarely learn to talk intelligently.

> Imbecile
> The *imbecile* may attain a mental level of six or seven years. Imbeciles can generally talk with a very crude vocabulary, can be taught simple manual tasks.
>
> Moron
> The *moron* ranges in mental accomplishment between the eighty-year level and the lower adult normal which is ordinarily reached at about the fifteenth year. Constituting more than 80 percent of all forms of mental defect, the morons are one of the serious problems of modern times. Having no gross physical defects, they present themselves as a shiftless, unstable group which gravitates to the lowest level of manual labor and social activity. Out of this class are the recruited, the petty criminal, the prostitute, and the ne'er-do-well."

In 1940 the idiot, the imbecile and the moron were *terms* that were *classifications,* and were not meant to stigmatize the individual. However, through the generational shift these terms were adapted as an insult to the "normal" public that did not apply themselves, or to basically devalue a person. The terms became so stigmatized that the mentally challenged and their loved ones divorced themselves from these expressions and advocated they are not politically correct. With effort, a new association emerged away from the idiot, imbecile and moron, and mental retardation (mild, moderate and severe) replaced the classification of these stigmatizing terms.

This is an important paradigm to examine when facing the prospect of de-stigmatizing a word imbued with devaluation. For example, the post idiots, imbeciles and morons did not wear a button stating, "I'm proud to be an idiot" or "Stop the stigma of idiots." They did not rally in masses at public parks, or stop people on the streets to explain that they are 'idiots' and educate the public that they are harmless. Rather, they removed themselves from any association of the words, and quickly. Now shifting from the idiot to mentally ill, how is it possible to reassign a new meaning that is politically correct for the mentally ill? How will the mentally ill divorce themselves from the 'sick puppies?" I suggest these questions are certainly worth considering since the mentally challenged used considerable intelligence to walk away from heavily stigmatized labels. The question now is, "Can the mentally ill do the same?" How much money and energy will be invested until we look for other less stigmatized terms? Consider the difference: "I am mentally ill" or "I have a chemical imbalance."

Stigma Soup

The chef that cooked up 'mentally ill' managed to make it a concoction that encompassed the reach of every synaptic threat against mankind, financially or dangerously. For example, the severely depressed is in the same stew as the pathological serial killer. We may see on the news wire, "A mentally ill pathological serial killer was found and arrested today in the wake of dozens of roadside murders" and in the same breath "...and in another local city a mentally ill woman perched high on a bridge stalled traffic until a crisis team was able to calm her and talk her down." The viewer of course, is introduced to the impression that the mentally ill is in the same pot as the poisoned serial killer. And, according to the "Diagnostic and Statistical Manual of Mental Disorders" (DSM), the psychiatrist handbook for assessments, that would be correct.

Physical Illness

Physical illnesses are usually addressed as a 'medical' problem and respectfully accepted as scientific in nature. These illnesses include cancer, cardiovascular complications and diabetes. There is much less stigma associated with physical illness. For example, we do not usually hear, "A physically ill serial killer was arrested today..." A physical illness tends to generate empathy and understanding rather than caution and avoidance.

Personality Disorders (not to be confused with deranged)

This is another interesting and confusing label. 'Disordered' suggests a defective personality structure at birth, when in fact may be very much 'ordered' in direct relation to the environment. I am suggesting the environment was disordered and the personality adapted to survive (effective). For every environmental ZIG, the surviving personality had to adapt and ZAG. The weaker and non-adaptive personalities (disordered) perished.

Authors and theorists, Otto Kernberg M.D. and Vamik Volkan M.D., to their credit realized the stigma of 'disorder' and referred to the DSM's Borderline Personality Disorder (BPD) as *Borderline Personality <u>Organization</u>*. This rings appropriate since the personality had to 'organize' defenses to survive. Those defenses are largely the result of a healthy response based on available and age appropriate resources at the time. The personality that is actually 'highly ordered' as a survival defense, is now stigmatized as disordered and lumped in with the serial killers as 'mental illness.' This categorical approach appears to put surviving personality as risk for stigma – a failure based approach.

Another interesting contradiction is that "Post-Traumatic Stress Disorder" (PTSD) is NOT viewed as a personality disorder but for the most part as a 'natural' and accepted response to a harmful environment, UNLIKE the closely related and stigma tagged survivor diagnosed with Borderline Personality Disorder.

DSM & Mental Illness

It is interesting that 'mental doctors,' authors of the 943-page handbook titled "Diagnostic and Statistical Manual of Mental Disorders" were also ambivalent about the book's title. They anticipated that the word 'mental' could have far reaching implications and this dilemma perplexed them as well. Yet, for the lack of more suitable word, 'mental' was adapted into the book's official title.

The adaptation of 'mental' is problematic because the brain is an organ (physical), and the mind (mental) is a complex of psych structures that are developed through life experiences. The brain is an organ with tissue as are other organs within the body. A statement that suggests the 'brain' is the 'mind' muddies the waters. Mental illness invites stigma that arises when the depressed individual (physical brain illness) is lumped into the serial killer psychopath (mental derangement). Is it any wonder the prefix "mental" is alarming?

Until advocates for the chemical imbalanced, i.e. bipolar, depression and schizophrenia (brain diseases) take a hard look at what is getting thrown into the same mixing pot with the (serial killers and child molesters), there is little or no chance to lift the stigma around "mental illness" as a brain disease. This is similar to a metaphor of mixing a few drops of red food coloring (serial killers) into a pot of water. The entire lot is now 'colored' as the mentally deranged. For example, it is highly unlikely that most parents would feel comfortable living next to a 'mental' person that is identified in the same line-up as the child molester.

Seventy-five years ago it was perfectly acceptable for a straight man to say, "I feel so gay today!" However, not likely nowadays!

Perhaps until there is a hard look at exploitation of 'mental' (DSM) that blankets across diseased brains, organized minds AND deranged minds, the stigma will remain.

Perhaps "mental" people and their advocates could learn a lot from the idiot, the imbecile and the moron. Only time will tell.

References:

Psychiatry for Nurses" by Karnosh and Gage (1940 - p. 237.)

Diagnostic and Statistical Manual of Mental Disorders - DSM-IV-TR

Borderline Conditions and Pathological Narcissism - Otto Kernberg M.D.

Six Steps in the Treatment of Borderline Personality Organization - Vamik Volkan

Regression

&

True Infantilism

What is True Infantilism?

Written by Kathi Stringer

Revision [N/A] July 31, 2002
Revision [E] June 21, 2007

Editor's Note:

The term ABDL is NOT True Infantilism. True infantilism is NOT about paraphernalia, or a fetish, or something to be practiced, props or costumes. The Term ABDL includes ALL of these terms as identifiers, whereas the term True Infantilism rejects these terms.

Introduction

There is remarkably little information on this subject. For this reason it may be helpful to establish a criteria to recognize true infantilism.

The onset of true infantilism is marked by earliest of memories fantasizing of regressive dependencies. Usually always during early childhood and youth the individual believed they are isolated and alone with their regressive desires, and that no one else in the world is like them.

These individuals for the most part keep their pervasive symptoms of needing to act-out the regression hidden from family, friends and significant others. A common theme revolves around wearing diapers, which in most cases will give rise toward a role-identification of an infantile personality. Over time the behavior in most all cases will expand to include other infantile objects such as pacifiers, baby blankets, baby bottles and soft stuffed figures.

Transitional Object vs. Fetish

A person may view true infantilism mistakenly for a fetish. There is a stark difference because the desire for the object occurred before puberty [2,4,5]. For example, the diaper may be regarded as a symbolic formation to ward of insecurities [4] and became a transitional object for a child [6]. In striving toward independence, personality fragments may fuse with objects that represented nurturing [7]. It appeared to provide a sense of control for the child to revisit a period that is widely accepted in our culture as nurturing. The energized transitional object offered relief from separation anxieties from the maternal figure and/or provided a sense of recreation for a period lost in grief.

The Abuse Connection

In some instances when abuse or neglect has traumatized a child [1], the small child may identify with toddlers in neighboring families and yearn for the same infantile attention. The child may secretly wish to exchange places and experience being diapered, cuddled, fed and nurtured as a renewed experience from a failed situation [8]. The observation of the attentive maternal figure construed as a representation for the unconditional love longed for in a healthy environment. This longing may become fixated in the individual's core developmental structures [3] because it provided a coping mechanism in absent of the good-enough mother. In essence, the fantasy of receiving infantile attention has helped the child survive and to emotionally refuel during a chaotic period. In most case these mechanisms will continue to manifest by way of recurring infantile fantasies through out the lifecycle of the individual.

The Libidinous Component

As the infantile child moved through the latency period in to adolescence, it is not uncommon for the transitional objects to remain with greater influence. After all, the infantile fantasy has been repeated many times along with its vicissitudes and is now firmly imprinted into the psychopathic structure. In some individuals, after the libidinous gratification component is augmented and integrated with the existing infantile fantasy, a new association emerges. The existing fantasy that provided a cathexis for emotional refueling is now set into motion with the more satisfying libido component. Essentially, the pre-libidinous transitional object takes on a new dynamic to relieve anxieties and to satisfy cognitive patterns set in childhood. It is not unreasonable to conclude that the fantasies imbued with the transitional object will become more concretized when intermittently connected to the libido drives.

Fragmentation and a Continuous Sense of Self

It is not uncommon for the infantile individual to become despondent from impinging feelings of guilt. After all, they may think that children do grow up one day and they have failed miserably.

Some infantile individuals tend to look at life as "all or nothing" terms. Either I am all regressed and unable to function, or, I am all grownup and must purge all the transitional objects. This thinking is much like a toddler uses in the defense of "splitting"[5]. A toddler relates to the world in all or nothing terms..i.e.."I love Mommy" or "I hate Mommy." A toddler is unable to tolerate conflict or ambivalence and it becomes unmanageable at times in the form temper tantrums because the anxiety ~~is~~ was too overwhelming [5]. In succinct, the infantile individual that is either engulfed with regression or defiant of infantile longings is behaving age appropriately with the toddler.

More desirable and because regression is an enduring imprint, it cannot be ignored. To bring infantile wishes in harmony with a higher level functioning, a comprise must be reached. This understanding of one's complexities will give way to a more continuous sense-of-self.

Dependency vs. Nurturing

Most infantile individuals incorporate a maternal figure into the childhood fantasy. This becomes a problem because to achieve a realistic experience the individual may seek out a mother figure and become depressed in her absence. It is for this reason I would like to point out a compelling difference between dependency and nurturing.

Dependency engenders neediness [3] and a notion that one cannot be nurtured without the presence of another individual. This is a false assumption that may lead to desperation. A belief that infantile expressions can never be meaningful unless dependent other others can be catastrophic. Dependency creates a dependency on others for happiness.

The infantile individual can nurture themselves with the advantage and use of transitional objects. The individual can simply be himself or herself and find happiness in being alive and able to experience regressive nurturing introspectively. An acceptance of self is the most nurturing aspect of life.

A Helpful Analogy

To concrete this a bit further. Transitional Objects, a term coined by Winnicott, is an object of attachment that the infant uses to provide relief. In true infantilism, a diaper is a transitional object from "earliest" memories....and holds a primary meaning of comfort and nurturing rather then a secondary sexual object.

This analogy may help to clarify true infantilism. A transvestite wears women's clothing for sexual gratification, and clearly a fetish. On the other hand a transsexual wears women's clothing from the desire to "become" a woman and some cases with Sex Reassignment Surgery (SRS) the transformation is complete, and this is not a fetish for a transsexual. I view true infantilism as more connected to the transsexual aspect of this analogy. In essence, for the true infantile individual, a diaper is not a fetish but rather a Transitional Object with its origins in early childhood.

Therapy and Treatment

There is no known cure for true infantilism. Its patterns and deliveries to satisfy infantile longings are set firmly into place. It appears to become problematic when situations place an emphasis for disclosure...i.e. getting engaged or getting married. The infantilized individual grapples for a decision because fears of ashamedness, rejection, abandonment and exploitation are commonly associated with past developmental struggles in childhood. It brings to surface a terrifying risk that a new partner or family member will misunderstand and take the position it is a bizarre perverted derangement and action to crush the behavior is paramount.

As stated, there is no known cure and treatment toward self-acceptance and individuality may ameliorate destructive wishes and behavior. Acceptance may resolve self-hatred and command the unrelenting forces of the cultural inner critic to subside. Because the personality is fused with the nurturing transitional object, in would not be therapeutic to destroy, purge, annihilate or defeat the mechanism that has provided some emotional stability for the individual. It would equate to most as wiping out the inner child.

One treatment modality may be applicable. A healthy balance is to be encouraged to help an individual from completely giving in to regressive behaviors. Introduce exercises to limit the fantasies to diminish pervasive regressive behavior since engulfment may create a larger abyss that is not grounded in reality.

Conclusion

I don't see how a therapist can help with regression, at least from my experience...unless; the therapist is there to help with self-acceptance and validation. Once one can accept self, then the forces are not so relentless...it can bring a feeling of...I am okay.... I am a unique individual and it is okay to be me. If an individual can accept that, then life can become more rewarding, and the inner child becomes loved. Each needs their own time. One should not starve the other, or put guilt on the other... individuals simply are they are

Written by Kathi Stringer and the essay "What is True Infantilism" may be reproduced with credits attached.

Reference:

1. Letter from Bruno Bettelheim 1978
2. The Transitional Space / Peter Giovacchini (p.28,80,81)
3. Prisoners of Childhood / Alice Miller (p.23,24,54)
4. Separation-Individuation / Margaret Mahler (p.108,157,171)
5. The Psychological Birth of the Human Infant / Mahler, Pine, Bergman (p.77,82,84,155)
6. Object Relations Individual Therapy / Scharff & Scharff (p.58)
7. The Facilitating Partnership / Applegate & Bonovitz (p.159)
8. The Language of Winnicott / Jan Abram (p.251)

BRUNO BETTELHEIM
ONE SIERRA LANE
PORTOLA VALLEY, CALIFORNIA 94025
(415) 851-2018

January 23, 1978

Dear Mr. Stringer,

I am writing you right away since I assume you are waiting for an answer. First let me assure you that your behavior is very understnadable, given your life history, although it is true that most ordinary people won't understand it. Be not afraid about having written me about it. I shall immediately destroy your letter, so that it can not fall into the wrong hands.

As you might know I am by now quite old and live here in retirement, no longer able to work. So, unfortunately, I can not help you personally

If what you do during the night provides you with relief you need, my advice is to continue with it, never mind what other people may think about it. Just keep it to yourself. The relief you give yourself during the night may well be what makes it possible for you to function during the day, and this is most important.

It is to be hoped, and it is reasonable to assume that this will be so, that when you fall in love with a girl who loves you and understands you, this will take care of your problems. Another possibility is that you seek treatment in some psychiatric clinic, but it will have to be one which is staffed by sensitive and humane persons. Unfortunately I do not know whether such a clinic is availbale to you where you live. But it might be worth your while to look into it.

The severe emotional deprivations you experienced in childhood makes it practically absolute;y necessary that you find something in your life that will compensate you for it. What you are doing is one way to do it. There might be other compensations which you may be able to find in life. If you do, you will no longer need to do what you are doing.

I am afraid that is all I can say or do. But I certainly understand very well why you are doing what you are doing, and I wish yo the very best luck for your future life, and that soon you will find some human being who will make up to you for all you missed, and then you wont need it any more. So take courage, things, I hope will turn up for you. This wishes you, your

Regression

Written by Kathi Stringer

Revision A - June 5, 2001

What is regression?

Regression is the return to an earlier developmental phase. Regression is also a defense mechanism. Winnicott (early 1950s) *"Regression is from genital to pregenital erotic experience of fantasy, or it is to fixation points belonging to the life of infancy in which pregenital fantasy is naturally dominant…typically, regression of this kind is from independence to dependence."*

What types of regression are there?

I will be discussing regression in *child alters* and regression as a life style. In the therapeutic environment I will be emphasizing on two types of regression, which are *benign* and *malignant regression.*

What is a Child Alter?

A child alter is the same as an inner child except for one major difference. An Alter is not integrated with the host and will not respond when 'called' back. For instance, if an adult is playing with a child, it could be said that inner child of the adult is also playing. But when the responsibility of the adult is summoned, the inner child will return and the adult can assume its role. However, a child alter may not return and continue to play. It is then an issue of communication. Some alters and the host are not aware of each other and in some cases and the host may lose track of time. Some dissociated persons may have alters that speak and help each other with communication or a co-opt system.

What causes regression or fixation?

It may be for a couple of different reasons. A person may regress when yielding to stress and return to an earlier level that provided satisfaction. Or a person may become fixated from trauma. For instance, an alter may be 2 ½ years old and its developmental phase arrested until integration can take place. Sometimes this is done through corrective parenting or *"reenactment."*

What is reenactment?

Reenactment is the conscious or unconscious wish to re-experience the trauma in hopes for a better outcome. This is commonly done in the therapist's office using psychodynamic therapy. *"This compulsion to repeat earlier trauma in present relationships* (the therapist) *is presumably based on an attempt to master the trauma through repetition with the hope of a better outcome, or, through a role reversal, to turn an enduring sense of passive defeat into active victory*" (Hedges 2000 – p.33, Terrifying Transferences). In order to recreate the trauma through regression in the office milieu, a therapist may use an interpretation tool called "*transference*."

What is transference?

Transference is the notions, conflicts and emotional investments that belong to a person from the there-and-then (past) and transferred to the therapist in the here-and-now. In all cases transference is a distortion. These feelings that are now attributed to the therapist are in some cases examined and interpreted for meaning.

What do you mean by "transferred" to the therapist? How is this done exactly?

It is usually an unconscious reaction in the therapeutic relationship. Note the following vignette I will cover transference, regression and reenactment:

> A 46-year-old patient that had a child alter that had a traumatic past with the mental health system was becoming increasing uncomfortable with her current therapist because of some of the material being uncovered (fear of intimacy, disclosure and criticism) in therapy. She was unable to link what was making her uncomfortable and suddenly announced that she was 'untreatable' thereby unconsciously avoiding the difficult subject matter in the present therapeutic relationship.
>
> Transference in this example works this way: The patient unconsciously '*transferred*' her notions and emotional investments from *past* failures of therapy and hospitalizations onto the current therapeutic environment to avoid delicate subject matter with her therapist. By labeling herself as 'untreatable', she attempted to dismiss the work in progress and sabotage the treatment in the here-and-now since prior treatment was traumatic and rejecting for her from the there-and-then. There is also a certain element of control in that the patient can sabotage the therapeutic alliance rather then wait for the expected impending doom based on past failures. In others words, "*I'll dump you* (transference from the past) *before you dump me* (as what happened in the past)."
>
> An astute therapist would grasp the impending dynamics and offer an *interpretation* as intervention. Notice that in this case we have a patient who had impulsed into regression – into the failures from the past. It could be said that patient used *transference*

as a vehicle and *regressed* in an unconscious attempt to *reenact,* hoping for a better outcome.

How would a therapist use interpretation in your last vignette?

In a continuation of the last vignette the therapist ascribes to Sandor Ferenczi's stance regarding treatability as Seinfeld (1993) elaborates, "*He protested against the idea of the untreatable patient and believed that any patient who asked for help should receive it, regardless of the severity of pathology. He asserted that if a patient was untreatable, it was because the analyst or analysis had not yet devised the necessary knowledge or effective means of intervention.*" In other words it was the method and not the patient that was inadequate.

Patient: "I don't seem to be improving and it bothers me that I am using up so much of the community resources. I'm just not treatable. Other people come in here and use the services and get better, but me, I feel like I am chasing my tail."

Therapist: "If you look at where you were a couple of months ago, you have improved."

Patient: "Yes, to a point. But I've been diagnosed as borderline personality disorder. I've read material that when a client isn't working, or able to maintain a relationship, both which involve complex people skills, that the chances are they are untreatable.... that is according to Joel Paris who writes for the APA."

Therapist: "But you have been able to work in the past and we have patients here that have made use of our services longer then you have. The services are here, and we are here for as long as it takes. I see that you are making progress and the other therapist on the treatment team sees that you are as well."

Patient: Long pause... "I don't know. I've been at this for so long and this writer Dr. Paris; he ascribes my symptoms as being untreatable. I don't think I should come back and just accept the situation as it is."

Interpretation

Therapist: "Do you suppose by any chance there is something deeper going on here? Perhaps you are unconsciously reenacting past failures with other mental health professionals? Now that we are making progress, it frightens you, that perhaps there are issues of trust and now you what to run. You fear that I will fail you like you've been failed before. It is hard work and there is bound to be instances that scare you, but we can and will work through them. Do you suppose this could be going on?"

Patient: I don't know, it could be. I know you are right, but it's so hard. I need to think about it…okay, I will keep trying and come again."

Hedges (2000, p. 202) *"…which helped me to see that she was successful in recreating her irritated mother with me, and that she was setting me up to reject her….I interpreted her terror in connecting with me and feelings of being abandoned, as well her attempts to irritate me enough so that I would leave her. She took in the interpretation and calmed."*

When should an interpretation be done and how?

Usually it would be prudent for a therapist to establish a strong *therapeutic alliance* and a good enough *holding environment* before attempting an interpretation since it could be seen as a criticism of the patient. In *supportive therapy* positive transferences are used to help institute the ideal therapist-parent. In other words, if the therapist reminds the patient of a person or object the patient idealizes, then a therapist may use that distorted transference to help build the therapeutic alliance for patient compliance. Once the therapeutic alliance is adequately intact the therapist may gently offer an interpretation. Seinfeld (1993 – p. 113) quotes Margaret Little on wording interventions, *"Winnicott often spoke tentatively or speculatively. Interpretations were offerings that the patient was free to accept or reject. Winnicott would say, "I think perhaps…" or "I wonder if…" or "It seems to me as if…" rather then make an authoritative statement."*

How is an interpretation therapeutic?

In our last vignette the therapist drew a parallel of past treatment failures into the present. In doing so the therapist was able to arrest early termination of therapy by the hopeless, frighten patient. In this instance, interpretation was therapeutic in that it prevented early dropout in treatment.

What do you mean by "holding environment?"

The holding environment is a term coined by D. Winnicott to describe the maternal and parental functions of the therapist. Social workers can especially relate to this term since their task mostly consists of empathically holding the patient through means of appointments with doctors, living arrangements, therapeutic support and problem solving.

Winnicott did not project the term to mean actual 'holding' which is all together impracticable with contemporary treatment due to liable risks and distortion. Applegate & Bonovitz (1995) *"Winnicott primarily employed the idea of holding figuratively."* Although it has been found that Winnicott did hold a patient's hand in particular sessions to calm the patient and give a sense of his being there. Lawrence Hedges comforted his patients in much the same manner (Hedges 2000 – p. 195, Terrifying Transferences) *"Her regressions initially took the from of an angry teen, a helpless child, and then a terrified infant. I sat next to her to help her stay present. Eventually, her regressions become so complete that only touch would help ground her."* However, Winnicott principally viewed the therapist's attention, support, interpretations, validations and empathy in the therapeutic milieu as "holding" to reassure the patient that he was indeed present in an atmosphere of protection and trust, hence the term *"holding environment."*

Could regression be a masque for repressed wishes?

Dr. Hedges (Hedges 2000 – p. 215, Terrifying Transferences) repeats a story that his friend Hedda Bolgar shares with him after she read *In Search of the Lost Mother of Infancy.*

> Hedda told a story of how years ago there was a woman who was wanting this type of contact or touch, and Hedda sensed that it was somehow very important for her. The woman was being seen in some sort of facility. Finally the woman was able to say, "I just want to sit on your lap and nurse." Hedda brought her a nursing bottle and milk and gave it to the nurse to warm (the nurse then thought Hedda was crazy!). As per the request, Hedda held her and let her nurse on the bottle. The woman was very happy. I believe this happened just once. The next day, she didn't need to be held, but still wanted to suck on the bottle. The following day, she said, "There is still something else that I want, but I don't know what it is." Hedda said, "I think you want me to promise that I will never leave you." That's what's behind so much of the yearning, that's what we all want. I had never heard that said so clearly and cleanly. In that instance, by giving her what she thought she wanted, the woman was able to express what she really wanted – never to be abandoned.

As we have seen in this vignette regression may indeed be acting out for a repressed wish.

What Is the difference between a benign and malignant regression?

The following explanations are aimed toward the professional's treatment milieu.

In a benign "therapeutic regression the patient seeks recognition" Seinfeld (1993) In other words he seeks to restructure his internal mechanisms for a psychic rebirth before the defective development took place, Seinfeld (1993, p.94) *"But from this regression the patient emerged much improved."*

A malignant regression takes the form of pleasure and gratification, rather then seeking internal structure change. It has the appearance of neediness while severely taxing the recourses of the therapist without making progress. A malignant regression takes on the illusion of satisfying preoedipal wishes of cuddling and tactile closeness when in reality a manifestation of gratification for genital libidinal strivings. Seinfeld (1993 – Interpreting and holding) recants Balint (1968) "*...the patient never has enough of his own needs met. As soon as a need or wish is satisfied, it is replaced by a new wish or craving, equally urgent. The regression in such cases resulted in an addictive state that was difficult to handle and often proved, as predicted by Freud, intractable.*"

What is a transitional object?

A transitional object is the love article of a child or adult that symbolizes some source of security. It could be in the form of a teddy bear, blanket, baby bottle, pacifier or diaper much like the baby blanket that the character Linus clung too in the comic strip "Peanuts." It belongs to the child and is unchanging and dependable. Usually the transitional object is soft and cuddly with a pleasant smell that signifies mother or primary caretaker. Wright (1991b) explains that *during the process of symbol formation, the space between infant and mother is filled by a transitional object that has the feel of the mother herself.*

As an infant becomes more aware of his budding new world around him, his awareness that mother is unavailable at times is more acute. The transitional object symbolizes mother and bridges the gap between dependence and independence and vacillates the transition. As the child begins to actively play, he assigns roles to play items and his ability to freely resign those roles to various objects moves in the direction of independence. Jan Abram (1997, p. 4) states "*Winnicott's discovery of transitional phenomena emerged from his appreciation of how the baby separated from mother and developed a sense of self. For Winnicott the capacity to use the transitional space represented the ultimate in human development and signified the ability to "live creatively" and "feel real."* And "*Winnicott saw the transitional object as the baby's real first true creative act, a bridge between the worlds of fantasy and reality* (Grolnick and Barkin 1978). Through repeated episodes of mother's absence, the child is able to tolerate longer periods of separations yielding to the transitional object. The transitional object is special in that it sets itself aside from other inanimate objects. While holding the object the infant differentiates between self and mother. David Levin (1985, p. 102) "*Here, from among myriad enticing and intriguing objects, a special, transitional object is found, one which will ultimately bridge the gap between self and other.*" The object soothes the child while the child is establishing independence during this 'gap', and realizes mother will ultimately return.

A transitional object for an adult may take the form of a medication prescribed by a doctor. The patient may feel more connected to the doctor taking the pills visualizing the doctor in a desired caretaker role. Winnicott (1959) *"…it is true that the transitional object and the transitional phenomena are at the very basis of symbolism."* It may even be a doll or other such object given to a patient by a therapist the help establish a presence when the therapist is unavailable. The patient may cling to the object until a crisis passes or to feel a sense of comfort. Seinfeld (1993) *"The therapist performing the holding function tries to provide the feel of mothering while maintaining for the patient the distinction that the therapist is not the actual parent."*

What is the difference between a transitional object and a fetish?

The difference between a transitional object and a fetish is that the love for a fetish is driven by sexual gratification or genital libidinal contentment but a transitional object helps satisfy an inner longing or emptiness. It is possible the object may serve both and create an internal unresolved conflict since the unusual sexual attraction is viewed as taboo. One may seek to disavow the taboo while clinging to the security of the transitional object. This may cause the individual to purge the objects while feeling a deep since of loss and confusion.

What is regression as a life style?

This case exemplifies how regression and transitional objects can merge into a life style.

The patient was born male and the oldest child in a family of four. He sustained great object and emotional losses during his childhood. His father was a prisoner of war for three years and brought the abuse home with him. The patient's mother left with the threat on her life when the patient was about 5-years-old and the father secured custody. When depressed, the father would drink, return home and terrorize his children by beating them or threatening them with weapons or torture. Other times his bad temper would flare and he would fly into a rage for no apparent reason and the children lived in constant fear. They were intermittently passed to foster homes or relatives and other times lived on the street without food for weeks at a time. The patient recalls the following incident:

> "Duepy, that poor kid. A terrified 2-year-old. We looked on in desperation as dad swung the rubber hose against his tender baby flesh. It was almost impossible to see the color of Duepy's skin through his swollen green, blue and black body.
>
> Again came the hose splitting the baby's flesh. We begged him to stop. Dad's face was red as it usually gets when he becomes worked up and out of control. He warned Duepy that he had better learn and stop forgetting how to put his pants on and now Duepy's

> biggest lesson was yet to come. We were instructed to build a bond-fire outside and heat water to a boil. "For what?" I asked. Then came the unthinkable answer. Dad planned to pour the scathing water over Duepy as punishment to motivate him to remember to pull up his pants. When the fire was built, I sneaked Duepy into the bathroom and helped him get his pants on. Duepy was shaking. He was so scared. His little eyes pleading for some intervention. Someone to protect him, to hold him, to love him. I tried the best I could to calm him so he could show Dad what a 'big boy' he was without tears. I knew the tears would just make Dad angrier.
>
> Duepy, a brave, beaten little baby pulled it together and showed Dad what a 'big-boy' he was by drying his tears and pointed to his pants – all pulled up. He must have been in so much pain with his swollen skin rubbing against those heavy jeans. For now, Duepy had a reprieve.
>
> As many beatings I have received from my Dad, I don't think none compared to how he beat Duepy day after day with whatever he laid his hands on. I don't remember seeing a smile on his face, only a look of fright and confusion. Thinking back, I do not remember Duepy's skin being free from welts or the shades of green and gray.
>
> At times I wonder what ever happened to Duepy, if he survived his developmental years. I wonder what affect the senseless beatings had on his impressionable mind. I wonder if he was able to secure any healthy attachments of trust. I wonder about Duepy, the baby that never was, only a 'big-boy'. I wonder....

During these traumatic years the patient would curl up nightly in the fetal position and enter into a fantasy that he had ideal parents. He imagined himself to be about 2-and-a-half-years-old, an age still in babyhood and yet able to express the autonomy of a toddler. It was only during these nightly regressions that the patient was able to drown out his core sense of deep emptiness. He sited this nightly ritual was his escape and used the fantasy to emotionally refuel from the harsh reality of the day. He carried his nightly regression with him into his twenties and became a very successful businessperson.

As the transitional objects became more and more a part of his daytime life, the patient became more disturbed over his behavior. He was afraid to share his 'secret' with anyone and visited the local libraries for clues to this conduct. He was able of locate two books, *The Empty Fortress* and *Love is Not Enough* by author and professor Dr. Bruno Bettelheim. He especially liked the book "The Empty Fortress" since the title seemed to relate to his empty-sense-of-self. He could relate to several of the books passages, particularly about one autistic child named Joey:

> ***The Empty Fortress***
>
> When we first met Joey he looked very small and fragile for his nine and a half years…what he so desperately longed for…sitting on his counselor's lap as she cuddled and fed him… Regression as Progress: While some autistic children wish only to have another babyhood and infancy of this kind, most want to be reborn altogether…Do these children somehow know that basic trust, on which alone we build satisfying relations to others, it best acquired during the infant's utter dependency on this mother, through the good mothering he receives? It is hard to believe they can know it, but something inside them must exert a powerful push in this direction, since they all want it so much and go to such lengths to recreate the situation…
>
> …. Only two dangers may be mention. The first is that the child may find the experience so comforting that he wishes never to leave it again. The more so because physiological developments no longer provide the push and support for the steps in personality growth. The chronology of physical and neural maturation is by that age out of gear with the structuring of basic personality and personal relations. Thus the task may seem beyond him and the child settles for being dependently cared for, the rest of his life.
>
> … Then the longing for infantile emotional experience may still induce him to be like a baby but with much of this armor intact… But there is also an entirely different type of regression: that of the adolescent who regresses out of deep inner need, or the regression we try to help our children engage in when the timing is right… Just because it is the most important progress the autistic child can make, the time, place and conditions for a symbolic re-experience of earliest infancy, if not life in the womb, must be his own spontaneous choice. It is essential safeguard against his permanent fixation at this way of experiencing the world… In short, he must have the conviction that his rebirth is self-chosen and self-regulated; that his development as a person from there on will proceed autonomously, with us as helper, not controllers.
>
> Even if we had had it in us to give Joey the infantile care he longed for, and without reservation, he could not have felt it that way. More likely it would have been one more case of being overpowered by adults… Though more then ready to give babying care under difficult conditions and to mean it, they were not ready to do this with Joey because they cannot meant it if the child does not respond a little humanly… We do not believe that total

dependent care does any good unless it is given with this conviction… For this reason we had to wait until Joey was ready himself. *But if he was to gather the courage, he had first to believe that good human relations were waiting for him to enjoy…*

Joey began to show more infantile behavior. It began with squirting water through the nipple of a baby bottle; he would not go so far as to suck from it yet. A few days later, he put a blanket around his shoulders and cuddled up in it. From now on for many months he was nearly always wrapped in a blankets covered up as he said, like a "papoose." Still he could only permit cuddling and other infantile care so long as he did not have to recognize them as such… While Joey wanted more and more to start life over, he could not comfortably anticipate another infancy in which he was totally helpless… He liked to put a towel between his legs as if it were a diaper, and to urinate and defecate into that. He called "playing baby."… *Activities once shunned were now attractive if they could be made in to symbols of infantile care…* Joey had long allowed his counselors and even Lou, his teacher, to hold him and carry him, had sat in their laps and let them cuddle him… On his own he let us know that now, after nine years (eighteen years old), it was time to leave us, and so he did.

A visit from Joey 3 years later:

Joey: There's a very interesting thing I was thinking of. I can remember the time when Fae and Barbara would feed me at the dinner table. Well, I remember having a much grater feeling of comfort whenever this happened.

Bruno Bettelheim (B.B.): When they fed you?

Joey: Yes

B.B. By hand?

Joey: Yeah

B.B. That was an important experience to you?

Joey: Yes it was.

B.B. Very good. When was this? Right at the beginning?

Joey: It was just a little after that. I think it started just before the anniversary of my first year there. And they also did it with baby food, starting the same time.

B.B. Where did they give you baby food, in session or at the dinner table?

Joey: They gave me the baby food in session and in the dormitory on my bed.

B.B. At night or during the day?

Joey: At night particularly.

B.B. And that made you feel very comfortable?

Joey: Yes, at that time....yeah.

Cont... B.B. So you wanted to start life all over again, is that it?

Joey: Yes, it was a way of starting life anew.

B.B. By then you were ready for that?

Joey: Yes.

B.B. Did you have such fantasies of being born again?

Joey: Yes, I did.

Joey had gone on to study electronics while working a part time job after he left the school headed up by Bruno Bettelheim.

After reading about Joey and several other of the children presented in the book "The Empty Fortress", the patient decided to contact Bruno Bettelheim. Upon contact the patient found that Dr. Bettelheim was already retired, but he promised to read a letter from the patient after a conversation on the telephone. With great anxiety and relief that patient wrote about his childhood abuse, the nightly regressions, the infantile transitional objects and infantile behavior. Within the month the patient received a response from Dr. Bettelheim. The patient recalled being terrified to open the letter fearing criticism and rejection but found quite the opposite and rather a wonderful empathic letter instead:

> January 23, 1978, Dear [Patient], I am writing you right away since I assume you are waiting for an answer. First let me assure you that your behavior is very understandable, given your life history, although it is true that most ordinary people won't understand it. Be not afraid about having written me about it. I shall immediately destroy your letter, so that it can not fall into the wrong hands.
>
> As you might know I am now quite old and live here in retirement, no longer able to work. So, unfortunately, I can not help you personally.
>
> If what you do during the night provides you with relief you need, my advise is so continue with it, never mind what other people may think about it. Just keep it to yourself. The relief you give yourself during the night may well be what makes it possible for you to function during the day, and this is most important.
>
> It is to be hoped, and it is reasonable to assume that this will be so, that when you fall in love with a girl who loves you and understands you, this will take care of your problems. Another possibility is that you seek treatment in some psychiatric clinic, but it will have to be one, which is staffed by sensitive and humane persons. Unfortunately I do not know whether such a clinic is

available to you where you live. But it might be worth your while to look into it.

The severe emotional deprivations you experienced in childhood makes it practically absolutely necessary that you find something in your life that will compensate you for it. What you are doing is one way to do it. There might be other compensations, which you may be able to find in life. If you do, you will no longer need to do what you are doing.

I am afraid that is all I can say or do. But I certainly understand very well why you are doing what you are doing, and I wish you the very best luck for your future life, and that soon you will find some human being who will make up to you for all you missed, and then you won't need it any more. So take courage, things, I hope will turn up for you. This wishes you, your
Bruno Bettelheim

Acting on Dr. Bettelheim's advice, the patient did seek help but was unable to make a connection with a therapist successfully. The patient continued the nightly regressions until his personality split into the "child" that he fantasized about. The child took on a life of its own in the form of a child alter (Dissociative Identity Disorder - DID). This alarmed the patient and he continued to seek treatment. He entered therapy for 3 months and then discontinued treatment since the regressions and the dissociative periods persisted.

In the patient's late twenties he entered into a program to change his sex hoping for relief. He reasoned that living as a female would be more acceptable to societal norms - that is, that childish behavior would be more acceptable in the female model then the male model. The patient did not disclose his present regression or dissociative episodes to the program director fearing rejection until the present problems were alleviated.

Once the patient entered into the program his regressive and dissociative symptoms began to subside. He attributed this to two reasons: 1.) the stress of the transformation distracted him from the regressions and 2.) his new feminine gender allowed an outlet for his babyish behaviors. Once the gender reassignment was complete her regressive and dissociative symptoms were held in abeyance for the next eight years. In 1996 her symptoms returned due to severe depression and high levels of anxiety from legal and other problems. She was hospitalized for dissociating for six days in her child alter state. Staff was repulsed by the regressive childlike behavior and tormented her with their cruel statements, inside jokes and punitive measures. This activated *post traumatic stress disorder* (PTSD) from childhood abuse and she slumped into a deeper depression and continued her dissociative states. During the next 5 years she cycled through severe depression, ongoing PTSD, Borderline Personality Disorder (BPD), DID and Bi-Polar Disorder with over 30 hospitalizations.

As of this writing, June 2001, the patient is currently in intensive therapy with a resourceful treatment team at Kaiser Permanente. She is working on her self-esteem and self-acceptance. Her goal is to integrate with her 2-and-a-half-year-old child alter and accept her childlike ways as a life style, and as she quoted Dr. Bettelheim, "*Never mind what other people may think.*" Her current M.D. Dr. Witkowski holds the same view and encouraged the patient with this statement, "*Who cares what other people think? So what if you are different. You are an individual. Just be yourself and you should be proud of being yourself, and that is what makes you an individualist.*" These words from her psychiatrist comforted her as much as Dr. Bettelheim's letter.

Summary

Even though regression may be viewed as a return to an earlier developmental phase, from the point of this work, it can also be a way of life. Through the use of transitional objects imbued with infantile strivings, an individual may be able to compensate for missing internal components. As Dr. Bettelheim suggested, there may be other compensations as well and once secured, an individual may no longer need the regressive behavior and transitional objects. However, the imprint may be to the degree that the individual may not be able to function without them. In such cases it is imperative to have a certain degree of understanding from family, friends and therapists to block deterioration of self-esteem, which can lead to self-aggressive acts observed in suicidal ideation.

The regressive behavior is harmless in the physical realm and usually the seat of the problem is in the attitudes of others. To withstand the pejorative stance in the community an infantile individual must have a clear sense-of-self and self-reassurance. An unstable personality structure can lead to self-loathing, depression and dissociating. A significant other or family member that wishes to change the individual with emotional pressure and confrontations will discover that it will usually backfire and results in repression leading to destructive forms of acting out. The individual may begin to withdraw affection, repress anger and frustration turning it inward on self or isolate from the 'badness of society'.

It has been noted that a transitional object is addictive, but it must be differentiated from self-medicating behaviors observed in alcohol and drug use. The object that is assigned meaning which soothes and comforts may be disturbing to a significant other that maintains the relationship should be sufficient without the need for a symbolic object or regressive behavior. Still, the individual's internal structures are already mapped through years of behavior and wishes and to change the mental organization would be much like trying to assign different connotations to the American Flag. To do either would certainly be met with resistance and distain.

Regression may also take the form of a child alter(s) known as dissociative identity disorder (DID). Some individuals may be able to integrate while others are able to maintain separation in a co-consciousness agreement through therapy.

In the therapeutic environment I have covered two forms of regression. The benign regression denotes reassignment of mental mechanisms and experiences toward a resolved sense-of-self through the therapeutic interplay of transference and projections, while a malignant regression presents itself as chronic neediness that fixates therapy. Once one need is gratified and new and similar need must be urgently met that severely taxes the resources of the therapist without the promise of improvement.

The Advanced Baby

Written by Kathi Stringer March 22, 2006
[Rev 1 April 19, 2006]

"Written by Kathi Stringer and may be reproduced and/or distributed on websites, and/or for personal use with the author's names and credits attached."

Imagine, in a world.... that for a few, age is timeless and innocence is for everyone that lives it, and growing up means growing smarter while daydreaming they are still in Carters. They can present with vestiges of adult maturity, while cloaking their infantile true self in the guise of adulthood. They may manage companies, formulate cooperate takeovers, and wheel the power to eliminate a division of executives. They may find themselves excelling to the top levels of their class, brainstorming ingenious formularies, or in the center of the party. They are frequently intelligent, progressive thinkers, spontaneous and creative. They can be found in classified and sensitive high-level operations within government, and all the while it is just a masque of a highly developed intellectual child. If you can imagine this, then hang onto your hat and get ready for a run around the Mulberry bush because it is quite possible that you've stumbled onto the elusive world of the advanced baby.

Ask yourself:

- Do you like snuggling up with a baby blanket or stuff toy?
- Do you bond with child-like friends with games like tinker-toys while cartoons are playing in the background?
- Do you feel like you cannot identify with the "A-word" – 'adult?'
- Do you like the baby-doll fashions, cartoonish clothes, or coloring in coloring books?
- Do you sometimes wear diapers and drink from a baby bottle as part of your identity?
- Do you feel comfort, loved and a sense of well-being from infantile associations of objects or play?
- Have you felt this way all your life and thought you were the only one?

If you can answer yes to most of the questions above, you may be an advanced baby, or suspect someone that is.

Introduction to the Advanced Baby – A Life-style

Just before the dawn of the new century, when Y2K was the hype, the term "Advanced baby" was coined to describe a life-style of infantilized persons. These individuals for the most part enjoy the grownup advantages of playing with computers and other high-tech gadgets with autonomy (= advanced), yet emotionally they still cling to infantile objects for security and comfort (= baby).

Phenomenon of the New Age?

Perhaps the phenomenon of the advanced baby is part of a larger spectrum that includes other groups of child-like individuals. Christopher Noxon, a writer for the New York Times, made a splash in the news circles after he articulated the occurrence of new terms in is editorial, **"I Don't Want To Grow Up**." *[1] In his article he uses terms,*

"Kidults, adultescents, or rejuveniles - call them what you will - the trend for immaturity is every-where. It has become unfashionable to be mature."

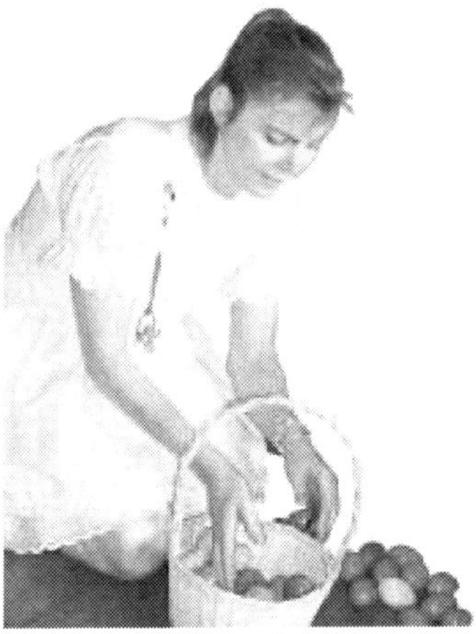

Noxon continued with an interview of Frank Furendi, a professor of sociology at the University of Kent at Canterbury in England. Noxon writes that Mr Furendi speculates that "adulthood as lost its appeal." Noxon writes further;

> *"Mr. Furendi began researching what he calls 'the self-conscious cultivation of immaturity' after spotting college students watching 'Teletubbies' in a university bar.* The scene stuck in his mind, and he came to think of it as representative of **a wave of infantilism** sweeping Britain and beyond."

Noxon's article caught-on and the mainstream of writers spurred further observation and speculation. Ian Shoales writes about the *"**World's***

Oldest Preteens" [2] that toymakers are targeting consumers that are buying products for made for persons half their age. Indeed, manufactures are considering another market for the infantile buyers. And, Trina Rea's article, ***"The Search of Eternal Youth,"*** [3] discusses 35-year-olds that are looking to escape financial demands in life by the attractiveness of regression. She writes,

"Is anyone surprised that they just refuse to grow up and are happy to regress back to childhood delights?"

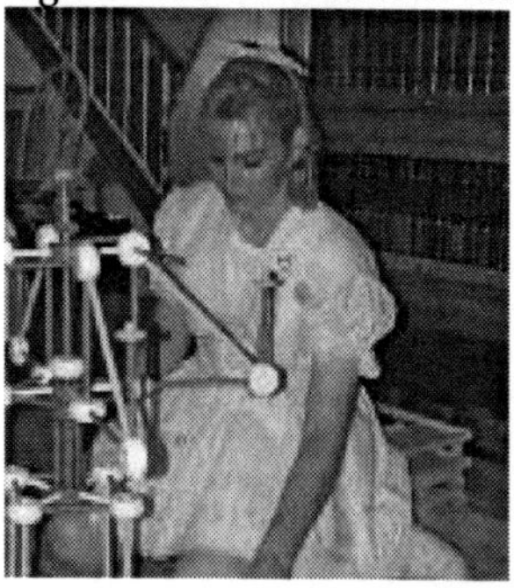

Rea indicates that it's big bucks for toy-makers and even publishers are jumping on the bandwagon and catering to *"Children's Books for Adults...Indulging rejuveniles - or kidults, as some are calling them. "* Siobhan McAndrew, from the Reno Gazette-Journal in her ***article I am a Gen-Xer suffering from Peterpandemonium***, [4] writes,

> "Others describe this back-to-babyhood boon as Peterpandemonium, Kidults and Adultolescents."

McAndrew indicates that is becoming a fad to wear knee-high socks and wear Strawberry Shortcake footed pajamas that now come in adult sizes. She echoes the New York Times that "Rejuveniles are not are not "stunted adolescents." They have "busy lives with adult responsibilities and respectable jobs."

Jessica Gresko, A Spectator Associate News Editor titled her article, **Stuffed Animal Attachments Carry Over into College Years.** *[6] Gresko writes about Andrea Herbst who admits bringing her teddy bear to college.*

> "*Dydee,*" *she got him when she was one year old.* "He came with the diapers from the diaper company," *she said.* "He has been with me everywhere. I took him to Germany when I was seven. He came to England when I spent the year there between high school and college."

Truly, we live in an age that older consumers are buying candy pacifiers, happy meals, and, according to Suzanne Fields author of **Revisiting the itsy**

bitsy spider, *[7] they* "don't want to leave their childhoods because they prefer innocence to edginess."

Advanced Babies and Defragmentation

The genesis of advance babies closely resembles their formation from the term "True Infantilism." [8] For most of their lives these individuals have had difficulty growing-up in the conventional views of adults. The advanced baby is not characteristic of being libidinally mature in adult relationships, nor are they indicative of even understanding themselves. Due to the unavailable information, it is an intangible-given that many appear to live in a world split by the "adult vs. baby" dichotomy. However, there is a conceptualization of a life without this dichotomy through a dialectical synthesis. Meaning a synthesis (= integrating the adult vs. baby) can reduce internal fragmentation to become a lifestyle to help an individual from completely giving in to regressive behaviors. The pseudo-adult and baby are defragmented and reflective of the true self.

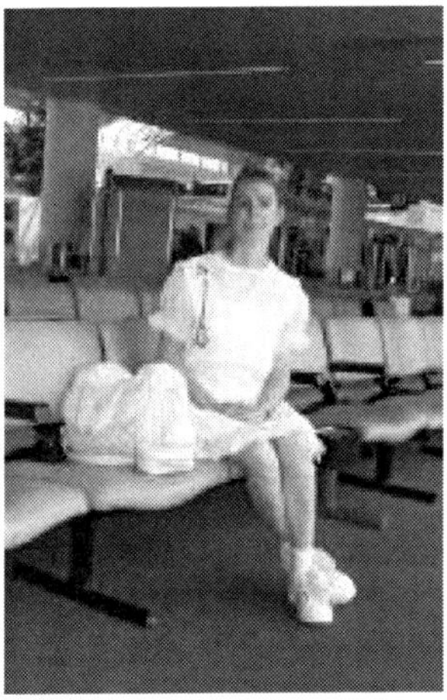

A Look at Transitional Objects – Not a Fetish, Costumes or Props

An excerpt from the essay True Infantilism [8] states, "A person may view true infantilism mistakenly for a fetish. There is a stark difference since the desire for the object occurred before puberty. For example, the diaper [or other object(s)] may be regarded as a symbolic formation to ward of insecurities and becomes a transitional object for a child. In strivings toward independence personality fragments may fuse with objects that represent nurturing. It appears to provide a sense of control for the child to revisit a period that is widely accepted in our culture as nurturing. The energized transitional object offers relief from separation anxieties from the maternal figure and/or provides a sense of recreation of a period lost in grief."

Transitional objects can carry over into adulthood and are often times not the original object. Glen O. Gabbard, the flagship author for the American Psychiatric Association indicates "Pills may function as transitional objects for some patients, allowing them to maintain some sense of connectedness with their psychiatrists when seeing them quite infrequently. Touching or looking at the pill may have a soothing effect on the patient." [9]

Advanced Baby – Self Identification

They've been this way most of their life from earliest memories. The concept of advanced baby is a lifestyle and is similar to the intellectual Peanuts character Linus carrying around his security blanket (term security blanket inspired by Linus Van Pelt) [10]. These behaviors are not viewed primarily as something to be practiced or a fetish. There is an important distinction to be made. There are many fetish and perversion sites on the Internet that assume to construct a comprehensive umbrella that state most regressed individuals fit into a their criteria using an alphabetical soup of acronyms. By making these blanket assertions, an individual is pigeonholed into a group with a range of behaviors that often appalls the listener (= countertransference problems). Often times, the infantile individual is horrified by the assumed associations and has no place to reference knowledge for treaters, family, spouses and friends. It's also problematic because it is not uncommon that an individual may wrongfully identify their personas with the contemporary slang on the Internet because they are not able to articulate it differently and nothing else is available. For these reasons, this essay on advanced baby has offered another option for self-determination and self-identification.

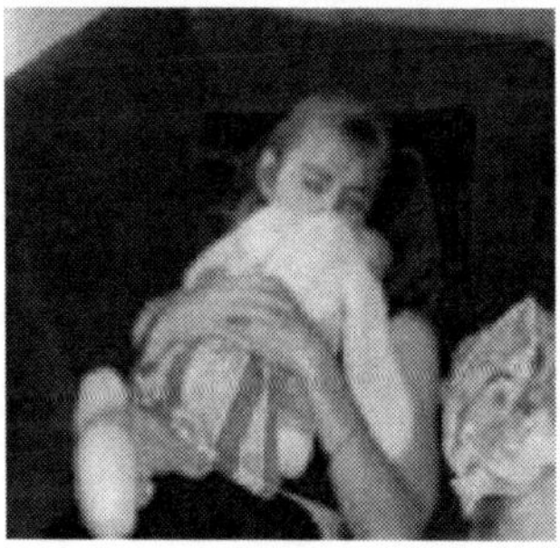

References:

1. Noxon, Christopher (Aug. 31, 2003***), I Don't Want to Grow Up!,*** New York Times. Extracted March 22, 2006, http://www.christophernoxon.com/nyt_sub_rejuveniles.html
Mirrored: http://www.toddlertime.com/dx/regression/notgrowup.htm

2. Ian Shoales (January 1, 2004) ***World's Oldest Preteens,*** Intelligent Enterprise Magazine, Extracted March 22, 2006
http://www.iemagazine.com/040101/701ddw1_1.jhtml?_loopback=1
Mirrored: http://www.toddlertime.com/dx/regression/youth.htm

3. Trina Rea, (December 19, 2003), ***The Search for Eternal Youth***, Europe Intelligence Wire. Extracted March 22, 2006,
http://www.toddlertime.com/dx/regression/youth.htm

4. Siobhan McAndrew (October 11, 2003), ***I am a Gen-Xer Suffering from Peterpandemonium***, Reno Gazette-Journal. Extracted March 22, 2006,
http://www.rgj.com/news/stories/html/2003/10/11/53893.php
Mirrored:
http://www.toddlertime.com/dx/regression/peterpandemonium.htm

5. ***Rejuveniles*** (2003-2004), Extracted from Kathi's Mental Health Review, Extracted March 22, 2006,
http://www.toddlertime.com/dx/regression/rejuveniles.htm

6. Jessica Gresko (November 14, 2002), ***Stuffed Animal Attachments Carry Over into College Years***, The Columbia Spectator. Extracted March 22, 2006
http://www.columbiaspectator.com/vnews/display.v/ART/2002/11/14/3dd38458acf7c
Mirrored: http://www.toddlertime.com/dx/regression/attachments.htm

7. Suzanne Fields (September 4, 2003), ***Revisiting the Itsy Bitsy Spider,*** Townhall.com. Extracted March 22, 2006,
http://www.townhall.com/opinion/columns/suzannefields/2003/09/04/168346.html
Mirrored: http://www.toddlertime.com/dx/regression/fields.htm

8. Kathi Stringer (2002), ***True Infantilism***, Kathi's Mental Health Review Extracted March 22, 2006
http://www.toddlertime.com/dx/regression/infantilism.htm

9. Glen O. Gabbard (1998) Psychodynamic Psychiatry in Clinical Practice, THE DSM-IV Edition, pp. 141

10. Charles Schulz (September 19, 1952), Linus, Meet the Gang.com Extracted March 22, 2006,
http://www.snoopy.com/comics/peanuts/meet_the_gang/meet_linus.html

11. Pictures for the advanced baby essay extracted from:
http://www.toddlertime.com/dx/regression/advanced-baby-pictures.htm

My Ideal Parent

Written by Kathi Stringer

Note: My treater asked me to write what I thought my ideal parent would look like. This was my response.

Shadowing and Darting Away

You would allow me to be close to you when I feel insecure. So that I know that I am loved when I feel frighten or helpless. In shadowing I could touch you to know that there is more then myself, and that you are an extension of me until I can grow into my own space. And then to test my limits of security, I may dart away only to be swooped up safely into your arms of peace and comfort. Yet, you do not engulf me and let me explore my world in the safety of your supervision. In shadowing and darting away I come to understand that there is stability in my life and that there is strength and protection beyond my own understanding. I feel loved and protected. I become confident and secure and curious about my new budding world about me. As time passes I am able to dart away in greater distances with security and confidence because of prior successes and familiar interaction with humanity, objects and things.

Separation-Individuation

During this development phase I take on the beginnings of being an individual and give up symbiosis and I test my surroundings as I separate into my own person. I watch your reactions when I connect to new experiences. I then take in your responses as a mirror refection of myself. This is how I get to know me a little better, through my reflection of you. As I become more individualized my new choices become more complicated and frightening at times. Yet you buffer my choices in the realm of your supervision and only allowing me choices that I am developmentally ready to make or accept. You acknowledge that as my own person, I grow developmentally different then others. In some places I may lag or accelerate depending on my own pace set to my personality and nature. Yet, because I am a beautiful child of the universe, I will continue to grow, when I am ready and my inner cup is filled with the needed ingredients. And because I am a developing individual, you do not compare me with other persons of my own age or likeness. You do not listen to peer pressure to contort my being, but rather instead allow our own personal experiences to shape my growth when I am ready, at my own rate. You give me time to develop into a wonderful loved human being so that I may find trust in the world.

The Good Enough Parent

Because you love me, you set a role model of me to follow. Since it is impracticable for you to be the perfect parent, you are by nature of love, the good-enough parent. At times when you slip or make mistakes, I notice the world is not perfect. It is these mistakes that prepare me for the real world of disappointments. I take them in one by one and give them meaning to shape my understanding of the world. Because you are the good-enough parent, I take on a realistic perception of my world around me. I learn how to enjoy the good moments and I learn how to prepare for disappointments.

Trust versus Mistrust

I learn about trust versus mistrust in that you show me the goodness of the world through your love to me. Through repetition of your loving good intentions I learn to trust and integrate a positive outlook of the world. You understand and endorse my primary need to be regarded and respected as the person I am at any given time, meaning my feeling of self, my core identity of emotions and sensations from my central sense of self. With trust you create an atmosphere of tolerance and respect so that I may develop in each phase and according to its own special ascendancy. You will not unconsciously assign roles for me to follow as a cathexis of your own unmet needs but rather allow me to bloom into the whole person I am.

Commonly Referenced Authors

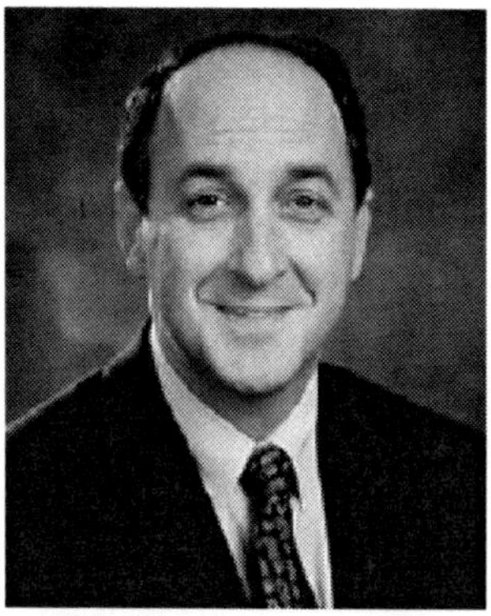

Glen O. Gabbard M.D.

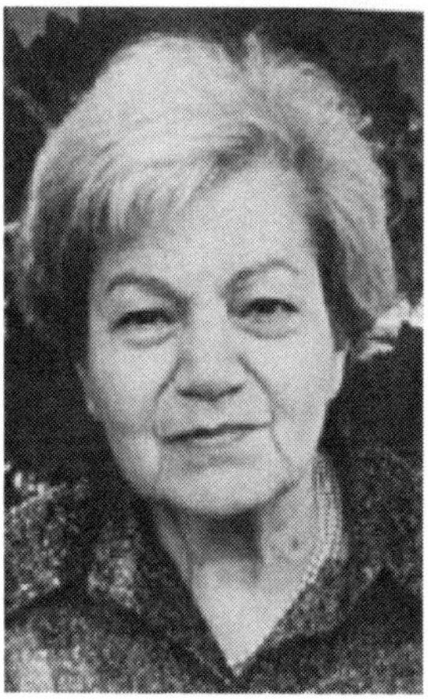

Dr. Margaret S. Mahler

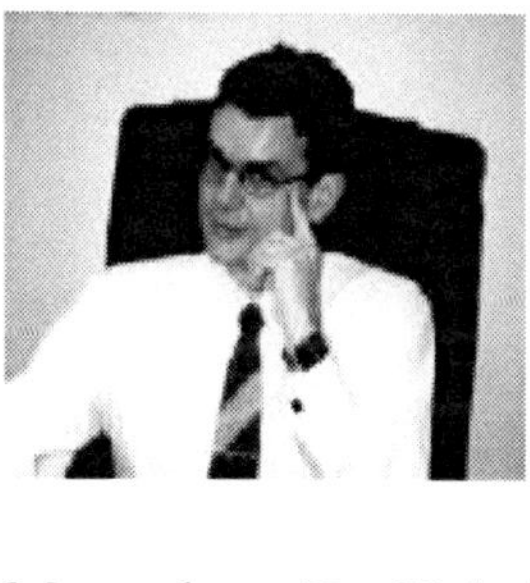

Sam Vaknin Ph.D.

More about Dr. Vaknin at the link below:
http://www.narcissistic-abuse.com/thebook.html

trust

Validation

Consistency

Constancy

Reliability

Strong therapeutic alliance

adequate conflict handling

p. 186 holding & containing

Lightning Source UK Ltd.
Milton Keynes UK
UKOW05f1910180713

214045UK00001B/102/P

9 780615 193137